# THE *Chemical* CONNECTION

LOUISE SAMWAYS

GREENHOUSE
PUBLICATIONS

First published in 1989 by
Greenhouse Publications Pty Ltd
122–126 Ormond Road
Elwood Victoria 3184 Australia



Cover and book design by Sharon Carr

Typeset in Australia by Solo Typesetting, South Australia

National Library of Australia
Cataloguing-in-publication data:

Samways, Louise, 1951– .
The chemical connection.

ISBN 0 86436 224 2.

1. Allergy. 2. Chemicals—Physiological effect. 3. Pollution —Environment aspects. I. Title.

616.97



Printed in Australia by Australian Print Group

# *Dedication*

To my grandfather, who instilled in all his family the confidence to say what you think and the courage to be different.

# *Acknowledgement*

All books are a lot of work and this one was no exception. It would never have been written but for my dear friend Dawn, who died before it was completed. Seeing it through was only possible because of the extraordinary patience, support and endless typing done by my husband John.

My young children put up with a mum often preoccupied and distracted by some hassle with 'the book' but cheerfully encouraged me just the same.

Lyn Timmons freed me from the practicalities of cooking and shopping so that I could get the first draft done in one stint.

My friend and colleague Judy Pledger provided a much needed professional sounding board as well as wonderful and unfailing support. And although I must take sole responsibility for the opinions and conclusions in this book the following friends and colleagues have at various times in my career given me an input of ideas or valuable support: Dr Ian Anderson, Neil Gilbert, Madge Parker, Joan Anderson, Geoff Wood, Dr Arthur Pearce, Dr Anwar Seedat, Jim Frew, Cheryl Couglin, Dr Colin Little, Dr Cees Van Tiggelen, Heather Robertson, Ingrid Scaramella, Janelle Chant, Sally Lee, Judy Peiris, Ros Orsino, Shirley Deane and the AAA Committees.

My two research assistants Graham Clue and Andrea Arranga were outstanding in their encouragement and help with computer searches of the literature.

Finally this book would be meaningless without the tremendous contribution, honesty and feedback from my patients and their families.

Louise Samways 1988

# *Contents*

It appears to me necessary to every physician to be skilled in nature, and to strive to know if he would wish to perform his duties, what a man is in relation to the articles of food and drink, and to the other occupations, and what are the effects of each of them to everyone . . .

Whoever pays no attention to these things, or paying attention does not comprehend them, how can he understand the diseases which befall a man?

*Hippocrates*

# *Foreword*

Louise Samways has written a very readable and thought-provoking book on the possible effects of some foods and chemicals, for all of us who have an interest in or are concerned about allergies and sensitivities.

For the lay reader, like me, this book gives some clear and helpful views about how many of the problems of behaviour and discomfort we all encounter one way or another in our lives may arise. The book is full of recognisable examples and situations, of a sense of the everyday, and of the variety of individual experience. Just those views and examples help to clear the air, and therefore may also help to remove some of the stress which, for families facing sensitivity problems, can compound their effects.

The book also offers some practical and understanding advice about how to avoid the effects of sensitivities, or at least cope with them, whilst making the very sensible point that it is best to consult a qualified health professional rather than self-prescribe.

I am also sure this book will stimulate discussion among health professionals. As its introduction explains, Louise Samways' background in psychology, her experience as an education guidance officer, and the familiarity she developed with nutrition and chemical environments, have together borne fruit in an holistic or ecological viewpoint. She is at pains to point out how a problem in one area, like a physical sensitivity not correctly diagnosed, can emerge in another—for instance in family relationships; she is also ready to issue a challenge to health professionals to recognise and treat such combinations of factors and effects. Whether they agree or not, I am sure the professionals will enjoy encountering her viewpoint.

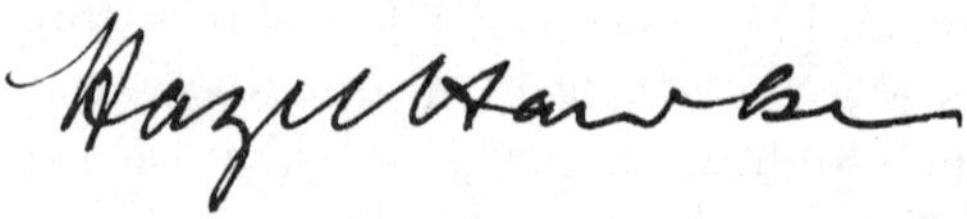

Hazel Hawke
Patron of the Allergy Association of Australia

# *Introduction*

'I'm tired, I feel awful, and I'm fed up with being told I'm perfectly healthy,' is the exasperated cry of increasing numbers of adults and children.

Health professionals are bewildered, puzzled and usually dismissive of such people as they come desperately seeking help.

But if you suffer from significant sensitivities to either foods themselves and/or chemicals found in your food, the air you breathe and the water you drink, you can feel just like this or have a multitude of other physical symptoms as well.

For instance, do you feel 'spaced out' or 'buzzy in the head' after using strong household cleaners on toilets and showers or when shopping in clothing stores or using photocopiers? Do you feel sick while having the car filled up with petrol or, alternatively, love the smell and can't get enough of it? Do you get headaches or ache all over after a day in the city?

These food/chemical sensitivities (some people call them allergies) occur when the body reacts inappropriately and therefore produces symptoms when it encounters a particular food or chemical in the environment.

So how did a psychologist end up treating patients with sensitivities and allergies? Why does a psychologist go into such detail about the physical features and indoor air environment of a home or workplace?

I am usually asked these questions by puzzled professionals, patients and the general public, particularly when I give lectures on food and chemical sensitivities. Interestingly, the general public can often see and accept a link between their emotional wellbeing and their physical environment much more easily than professionals.

To understand the context and perspective in which this book is written, it is necessary to understand my own background and experience.

After graduating in Science (Psychology and Genetics) I completed a Diploma of Education. I then taught science for two years in a secondary school. Two years of teaching experience was a prerequisite for transferring to the Counselling Guidance and Clinical Service Branch of the Education Department of Victoria where I undertook three years of clinical training and supervision to become a psychologist. For the next four years I worked as a Guidance Officer. My work involved consulting in normal schools and kindergartens, and in schools for retarded children. Apart from counselling and clinical work with children and their parents, a great deal of time and training was devoted to intellectual assessment and the diagnosis and treatment of learning difficulties. These assessments were usually made in schools and homes where the physical conditions were often appalling.

During this time I visited literally hundreds of homes and over fifty schools and kindergartens where either the children, adults, or both, had emotional or learning difficulties.

The Southern Mornington Peninsula Area where I worked for much of that time had been traditionally a seaside holiday resort area with a low permanent population. A large part of the Peninsula was rural with orchards and market gardens which were heavily sprayed each year.

With the increasing divorce rate and high rents in Melbourne this area was now attracting large numbers of single parent families and financially stressed families as cheap rental accommodation was available for most of the year. Unfortunately, much of this rental accommodation consisted of holiday houses which were not built for winter climates, and often did not comply with building regulations. Many were little more than shacks or converted trams, buses etc. A number of families lived 'temporarily' in old wooden caravans or sheds while they built their homes over months or years. For others the situation was permanent.

This experience gave me a unique opportunity to see differences in behaviour of the same patients under vastly different physical conditions. Teachers described one child as looking 'hungover' each morning but after morning recess he was described as 'no problem', although the teachers still felt he was not working to his full ability.

His mother described him as aggressive and uncontrollable at night, with nightmares most nights. From the interviews with the mother and teachers at the school I initially assumed some problem with the mother's management of the child—until I visited the home, a common procedure in this rural area. The house was little more than a shack made from cement sheet and corrugated iron. It was bitterly cold and overhung by thick tea-tree and a pine tree which cut out the light and sun most of the winter. The house smelt mouldy and in fact there was visible mould on the walls and ceilings. The only heat was a very smelly kerosene heater. To keep warm the family lived in one room and kept all the windows and doors shut. The mother said that since moving there she had developed migraine and asthma but described her life as, 'better than in Melbourne', as she had left her very violent husband. She reported that in Melbourne her son had always been extremely placid and his temper outbursts were frightening her a great deal. He hated his father and she very much doubted that he was now, 'assuming his father's role', as I rather meekly suggested. After each visit to this house I felt quite ill myself, so I decided the best 'therapy' might be better housing. After using my contacts to find this mother a job, she was able to move. Her migraines disappeared and so did the child's nightmares. The child was no longer 'hungover' at school.

This family's home was typical of many I visited and my strongest memories of these home visits are of the darkness, the smell of mould and the kerosene heaters.

As a result of this very demanding and often frustrating work I began to wonder whether there were physical factors (eg: indoor air quality) influencing behaviour that were not being adequately considered.

Many of the children (and the parents) I was seeing had a multitude of minor and sometimes major physical symptoms as well as psychological problems. Both doctors and psychologists tended to dismiss these symptoms as functional or just 'something problem kids tend to have'. The paediatricians and general practitioners to whom I referred patients kept telling me that despite their symptoms the children were 'quite healthy'.

To me, there appeared to be numerous subclinical and frank clinical symptoms (sleep disturbances, repeated infections, rashes, stomach pains, chronic diarrohea or constipation) being ignored or put down to 'nerves'.

During my home visits, I also became increasingly concerned with diet and nutrition. The more questions I asked about family and children's diets, the more alarmed I became. It was not uncommon to see children who were consuming the equivalent of sixty teaspoons of sugar each day hidden in their food and drinks. Commonsense suggested some changes in diet. Even quite simple dietary restrictions avoiding additives and sugar often produced dramatic improvement in behaviour—particularly in activity levels and aggression. I became puzzled however by the deterioration in behaviour and increase in physical symptoms when certain patients 'improved' their diet and increased their consumption of milk and whole grains. It was apparent that some so-called good foods were very bad foods for some people—'one man's meat is another man's poison'. This rather confusing phenomenon made me realise that good nutrition was not enough—unusual reactions to food had to be considered also.

At times I felt quite angry at the emphasis on the parents' (usually the mother) or the teacher's shortcomings—even when the parents had other perfectly well adjusted children and the teacher had an outstanding record with model classes. If no really major physical reason (eg: birth trauma) could be blamed then the parents and school became the scapegoats no matter what the problem—from soiling to aggression to learning difficulties.

I considered the possibility of chemical sensitivity further when a very active little boy with major learning difficulties and night terrors was referred to me. Throughout the interview he constantly fidgeted, plucked and pulled at a shiny synthetic tracksuit he was wearing. To my casual observation the tracksuit was irritating him and I quite innocently asked the mother if he wore it often. I was surprised to hear that he had virtually lived in tracksuits (including sleeping in them) since he was a baby, as his aunt worked in a clothing factory and the family could buy 'seconds' very cheaply.

I suggested they borrow some natural fibre clothes if necessary and keep him out of tracksuits for a week—letting him sleep naked if they could not afford cotton pyjamas. Frankly, I didn't expect any significant change but the list of problems the family had was so long and the mother felt so hopeless I felt it was something concrete for her to do until I could arrange for a social worker to help with the socio-economic difficulties.

I was greatly surprised to receive a phone call a few days later to say 'Bobby was fixed'. Apparently within twenty-four hours of changing his clothes his night terrors stopped and over the next few days his activity level became more normal. The tantrums ceased and severe bouts of aggression had stopped. The mother reported that they felt like I'd given them a new son. Unfortunately the family moved again not long after so I lost contact but the teacher who taught Bobby for a few weeks before they moved said she was astounded at the transformation in his personality and concentration.

After these experiences I was relieved to read two books which made me realise I was not imagining my observations—*Pychodietetics* by Dr E Cheraskin and *Not All in the Mind* by Richard Mackerness.

After leaving the Education Department in 1979 to have my first child I had no intention of returning to work for some years—if ever! However a few of my former patients contacted me, wanting follow up, and a few weeks before my daughter's birth I found myself rather reluctantly in private practice.

Since then I have been in private practice specialising in the areas of clinical nutrition and clinical ecology.

In late 1983 Dr Colin Little, Director of the Allergy Unit at Bethesda Hospital, asked me to work with him, specifically to help in the diagnosis and management of allergy/sensitivity patients suffering psychological and physical symptoms. This enabled me to further observe and test changes in patients' intellectual performance and mood when exposed to various foods and chemicals.

This book is based on my clinical observations and test results over the last ten years. At one time I attempted to conduct some research in conjunction with the Psychology Department of La Trobe University. I soon realised that the emotional commitment and time restraints of having a family and running two clinical practices made it impossible for me to conduct research myself. I decided I would have to restrict myself to clinical practice, and encourage others to undertake research.

This book is in response to requests by colleagues, patients, teachers and doctors who wanted to understand and minimise this alarming problem of food/chemical sensitivities, which is usually completely misdiagnosed or ignored all together. To achieve this, I and a group of colleagues and patients have set up the Allergy Research Organisation of Australia (AROA) which is a Federal Government approved research institute.

Although much of this book describes extreme situations and case histories to illustrate a point, the effect of food/chemical sensitivities vary on a continuum from slight to overwhelming symptoms. Whenever I have spoken to large professional and public audiences over the years, I have been very surprised to find that most people can relate immediately to the symptoms and situations I describe, suggesting that far more people are being affected than I ever suspected. The group of patients I see appear to be the extreme end of a much larger problem. The question doesn't seem to be whether a person is sensitive or not, but *how* sensitive.

When testing I have found that patients often show dramatic deterioration in reaction times and increased distractibility after even minute exposures to single chemicals. This is rather worrying when you consider the degree of chemical exposure people receive when driving from both inside (plastic and vinyl) and outside (smog) the car.

The 'I feel like I'm getting the flu' feeling is a very common symptom of sensitivities. The aches and pains of having the flu come, not from the bug itself, but from your body's reaction to it—your immune system is on full alert and ringing alarm bells throughout the body.

Patients report feeling that they are being robbed of the 'joy of living'. They feel out of contact with their emotions. Life experiences seem muffled by a 'heavy fog'.

Children are at greater risk than adults as their bodies and central nervous systems are still developing. Satisfactory social, emotional, and intellectual development depend on an 'intact' nervous system. Children are being exposed to the same chemicals as adults but their body weight is much smaller and their metabolism much faster. They are physically closer to such hazards as dusts and flooring materials (eg: glues in carpets, foam carpet underlay) etc. This is a problem particularly if the floor is heated.

*This book does not pretend or intend to be a conclusive document on the effects that food/chemical sensitivities can have on behaviour but rather intends to stimulate interest and research by those in a position to do so and to create a better understanding by those in the helping professions of just how insidious and profound the effects of food/chemical sensitivities can be on intellectual performance, educational achievement, and social and emotional development.*

The consequences of sensitivities for the community are frightening and can be catastrophic for those badly affected. Psychologists may be forced to review the reliability of many common psychological tests. Architects and builders will need to question the materials they use, educators will need to look not just at the students but at the physical environment in which they teach and what the students are eating. Doctors and psychologists will need to review their diagnoses of functional complaints. Government departments *must* review health legislation. If this book stimulates a questioning attitude in my colleagues in the helping professions, and in our long-suffering patients, then I feel it will have achieved its aim.

Those not presently 'sick' need to recognise that food/chemical sensitivity is an insidious problem affecting us all to varying degrees. The sheer numbers of unknown chemicals now in our food and air, not to mention the interactive effects of this brew, make it practically impossible to research the effect of these chemicals individually on behaviour.

In the 1980s our home, school and work environments have indoor air which is a chemical concoction producing 'pickled people'—our bodies and minds are being shrivelled and distorted in the process.

This book explains how this is happening, the consequences, and how individuals can minimise the effects on themselves and their families.

# PART ONE

# *Food/Chemical Sensitivity and its Role in Behaviour*

# CHAPTER ONE

# Ecological Model of Behaviour

Over the past decade the phenomenon of food/chemical sensitivities has been recognised by a small but increasing number of medical health professionals, natural therapists and lay people.

From my own observations over the past ten years I would estimate that at least a third of the children in Australian schools are having their educational achievement and social and emotional development significantly affected by food/chemical sensitivities.

These clinical observations are making increasing sense in the light of recent research on a biochemical/molecular level. Although there is much clinical and

* *If you haven't read the introduction because you think all introductions are boring and irrelevant then go back and read my introduction now! In this book the introduction is important in understanding my perspective and the context in which the conclusions and observations in the following chapters are made.*

increasing amounts of scientific evidence for food/chemical sensitivity, there is still not a lot known about the mechanisms through which food/chemical sensitivities occur and how they act to affect behaviour.

The terms allergy and food/chemical sensitivity are often interchanged causing enormous confusion and argument between lay and professional people. The effects of foods and chemicals on behaviour are highly unlikely to be due to traditional allergic reactions. The behavioural effects are more likely to be due to other kinds of inappropriate immune response or other mechanisms entirely.

Therefore, before discussing how food/chemical sensitivities can effect behaviour it is necessary to define a few terms.

## Allergies

Throughout this book I use the term 'allergy' when speaking of 'traditional' allergies.

Traditional allergic reactions are well known to cause eczema, asthma, hayfever and skin rashes—referred to as atopic symptoms.

The reactions are mediated through a system called an Immuno-globulin E response, resulting in the release of an inflammatory substance (eg: histamine). Symptoms usually arrive quickly, peaking after approximately fifteen minutes and lasting for about two hours. They may involve itching, redness and wealing of the skin. Large quantities of mucous may be formed within the air passages and digestive tract.

## Sensitivities

The term food/chemical sensitivity is used for symptoms which may arise from other inappropriate responses of the immune system, or by any other as yet unknown mechanisms.

**Behaviour**

There are library shelves full of books attempting to define behaviour. For our purposes we will define behaviour as anything a person says or does that we can observe and usually measure in some way, eg: rate of speech, time spent sleeping, mood changes etc.

Behaviour should be seen as the end result of a complex interaction between many systems within the body. The body aims for a state of homeostasis (stability). To achieve this, pressure on one system may be compensated for in many other systems of the body in a complex bio-feedback mechanism.

Many systems may in fact be stressed for some time before obvious changes in behaviour or symptoms occur— for example, you may be thirsty before you actually change your behaviour and seek water, or become irritable or nervous before developing a headache or other physical symptoms. All parents are familiar with the irritable child who later breaks out in spots!

It is important to realise that behavioural changes are much more likely to be observed well *before* physical symptoms occur.

# * Ecological model of behaviour

In this book and in my clinical practice I take the view that behaviour and behavioural symptoms must be seen as the outcome of an interaction between emotional and physical factors in an individual's internal and external environment.

---

* *Ecology: Study of the relationship between animals and plants and their surroundings.*

**EXTERNAL**

| | | |
|---|---|---|
| | FACTORS 1 | FACTORS 4 |
| | Peers | Light |
| | Family | Air |
| | Work/school | Chemicals |
| | Community | Humidity |
| | | Moulds |
| | | Electromagnetic |
| | | Radiation |
| **EMOTIONAL** | | **PHYSICAL** |
| | FACTORS 2 | FACTORS 3 |
| | Self—Personality | Genetic |
| | —Feelings | Congenital |
| | —Perceptions | Disease States |
| | | Physiology |
| | | Nutrition |
| | | Allergies/ |
| | | Sensitivities |

**INTERNAL**

# The four groups of factors within the ecological model of behaviour

## Factors 1—The External-Emotional environment

This refers to the environment in which individuals live their life, and which influences their thoughts and belief structure. External–emotional factors include events within a person's family, peer group, school and/or work place, community and society at large.

## Factor 2—The Internal-Emotional environment

This involves an individual's personality—his or her thoughts, perceptions, emotions, feelings, moods and beliefs.

The interdependence of the external-emotional and the internal-emotional factors is probably the most obvious within this model as there is a very clear interaction between them. External-emotional factors affect a person's emotions, thoughts and feelings, and likewise a person's thoughts and ideas affect his or her perception of the environment. This area, involving the emotional and psychological functioning of the individual, has been primarily studied and treated by psychiatrists and psychologists.

## Factors 3—The Physical-Internal environment

The physical-internal environment of a person includes congenital factors, genetic conditions, allergic reactions, nutritional and physiological states (eg: endocrine and nervous system functioning) and disease states. These factors have been traditionally dealt with by doctors.

## Factors 4—The External-Physical environment

Until recently this factor was given very little attention by any group of health professionals. Light quality, air quality, the composition of air (eg: the amount of oxygen in the air compared to carbon-dioxide) and air temperature are all features of the environment which can affect behaviour. Chemical contaminants in air, food, water and housing are being increasingly considered as potential health hazards. Electromagnetic radiation is also considered another probable hazard.

In Russia, light quality and its effect on behaviour has been studied since the 1950s. Miners in Siberia spend long periods in mines. During the short Arctic winter days, they are only exposed to very small amounts of natural daylight. This was found to create a range of behavioural symptoms such as moodiness, depression, anxiety and irritability which were alleviated when the exposure of the miners to natural light was increased artificially.

A recent American study observed the effects of light quality on activity levels of both children and teachers. When ordinary flourescent tubes were replaced with 'Daylight tubes' (a wide-spectrum light band), significant changes in the activity levels of both children and teachers were found.

Another study has shown that full spectrum flourescent lighting in the classroom dramatically reduced school absences through illness suggesting a direct effect between light quality and the immune function.

## Analysis of behaviour problems using this model

**Example: Sleep Problems**

Sleep disturbance is one of the most common reported behavioural symptoms. Using this model one can see that whether you get a good night's sleep or not depends on a whole range of internal and external, emotional and physical factors:

| | |
|---|---|
| Factors 1<br>External-Emotional | —fight with boss at work<br>—fourteen-year-old daughter wants to go on the pill |

| | |
|---|---|
| Factors 2<br>External-Physical | — jackhammer on road at night outside bedroom window<br>— bed lumpy<br>— cold<br>— partner snores |
| Factors 3<br>Internal-Emotional | — scared boss will sack you<br>— worried daughter will get AIDS |
| Factors 4<br>Internal-Physical | — sleep apnoea (A sleep disorder<br>— in which a person cannot breathe properly and is starved of oxygen.)<br>— hungry<br>— twelve cups brewed coffee drunk during the day |

Unfortunately, sleep problems and other behavioural symptoms are rarely assessed or treated in such broad terms in practice.

Patients tend to be divided into 'pieces' by professionals with the result that each professional has a piece of the jigsaw but often can't see the complete picture.

From my clinical experience and from the increasing research into environmental factors affecting behaviour, I believe behavioural symptoms must be diagnosed, assessed, and treated considering all four groups of factors.

## Problems of diagnosis

Labelling is not a complete diagnosis. Labels simply name symptoms. A complete diagnosis not only names symptoms but identifies the causes which then suggest treatment options.

For instance, for twenty years hyperactivity has been a much discussed phenomena in the scientific and popular literature. But there is now increasing wariness regarding the reliability and appropriateness of labelling children as hyperactive (or, alternatively, as having an 'attention deficit disorder with or without hyperactivity').

The trouble is that all the symptoms considered to be those of hyperactivity or attention deficit disorder are also found in varying degrees in other childhood disorders, eg: autism, childhood psychosis, organic injury, genetic problems, intellectual retardation.

The ecological model can often be used as a more productive way to treat children (or adults) exhibiting symptoms commonly put under the hyperactive umbrella such as impulsiveness, irritability, hyperactivity, learning difficulties, aggressiveness, socialisation problems, contrariness, stubborness, etc. etc.

From a research and clinical viewpoint it can be a waste of time to conduct endless tests, interviews, and observations in order to come up with a 'label' euphemistically called a diagnosis. In the medical and helping professions, accurate diagnosis is usually considered crucial for appropriate treatment. Ideally, diagnosis should include an understanding of the *reasons* (which may be multiple) for the symptoms. However, labels often hinder rather than help that understanding. If labels were put on causes rather than symptoms, research might move a lot faster and be more relevant to patients' needs. Unfortunately, diagnosis too often stops at labelling, which may make the professional feel rather clever but may not help the patient and his or her family.

By looking at labels not symptoms, the practitioner can conveniently disregard symptoms that don't fit his or her label. Most patients do not come to consult me until they have 'tried everything else and been everywhere'. These patients have been put in the 'too hard basket' by other practitioners because their symptoms won't conveniently fit traditional labels. Many patients in this situation silently suffer and just keep quiet about the symptoms that don't fit. They let the doctor treat what does fit a label in textbooks and try to pretend that the others don't exist.

More persistent patients who demand answers often get labelled 'difficult', 'neurotic' or 'obsessive'.

The ecological model of behaviour attempts to look at the possible causes for symptoms. Just as there are multiple symptoms of, say, 'hyperactivity' or 'attention deficit syndrome', there can also be multiple causes which require accurate diagnosis and treatment by a multi-disciplinary team.

## Possible factors contributing towards typical 'hyperactive symptoms':

| | Internal Factors | External Factors |
|---|---|---|
| Physical | Organic<br>—genetic defects<br>—mental retardation<br>—trauma (head injury, infection)<br>Functional<br>—allergies<br>—EOS dysfunction<br>—hypothalamus dysfunction<br>—nutritional deficits and nutritional bioavailability<br>—pharmacological eg: drug effects<br>—muscle/skeletal problems | Chemical in food/air/water<br>Temperature<br>Humidity<br>Light<br>Electromagnetic Radiation |
| Emotional | Self<br>—personality<br>—self-esteem | Family<br>Peers<br>School<br>Community |

It is most important to be aware that symptoms are produced and modified by a dynamic *interaction* of these factors. All factors must be considered together and priorities for treatment based on how interactions will affect the dynamic picture.

Imagine a house of cards where the house is the symptoms and the factors creating the symptoms are the individual cards. Some cards will be more crucial than others to the overall structure. Some houses (symptoms) can be dismantled quickly by removing one crucial card (factor); others will need to be tackled more slowly and methodically depending on the patient and his or her emotional resources.

Unfortunately, there is often a tendency to focus on particular symptoms with no consideration for the consequences for the patient. This is commonly seen with depressed patients who have been on long-term anti-depressants, presumably to stop them suiciding. As one patient put it—'On anti-depressants I no longer want to kill myself but the side effects of the tablets make my life not worth living.'

Similarly, parents with a 'hyperactive' child reported that drugs like Ritalin 'make him bearable to us but make life unbearable for him'. (However, it must be noted that drug therapy can be extraordinarily successful for some patients and their families).

The ecological approach demands multidisciplinary teamwork and this means that professionals must be prepared to gain insight and knowledge about what other professionals can offer to patient care and research. Although many people profess to believe in multi-disciplinary approaches (holistic healing etc.), in practice there is a rather indecent grab going on for the patient dollar so that referral outside a private practitioner's own profession is still very unusual.

Doctors tend only to refer to other doctors or psychiatrists; psychologists tend to refer to social workers or another psychologist. There is often not a great deal known by the helping professions about where each of the other helping professions can assist, and there is sometimes resistance to referring patients on to others. In my experience this can be very detrimental to patients. For long-term success with behaviour problems, all four interdependent factors—that is, the external and internal emotional and physical factors—must be at least considered, weighted appropriately and then treated in the right order. Sometimes the problem will be mainly physical in which case a physical or medical type treatment may be sufficient. Often the behaviour problem will exist largely due to psychological/emotional factors, in which case psychological treatment will probably get the best results.

Sorting out which is the most important factor, or in which order factors should be tackled, are very complex issues. When looking at behaviour problems professionals need to be aware of what other variables may be contributing to the symptoms, often outside their own area of expertise. For instance, psychologists need to be aware of the physical-internal factors which may affect behaviour; doctors need to be aware of the emotional factors that may be operating, and so on.

As our society becomes more technologically sophisticated and the chemical contamination of our world increases, it is becoming increasingly necessary to look at all four factors and treat a behaviour problem as one with the potential for four complementary solutions.

I am not suggesting that food/chemical sensitivities are the sole cause of all behavioural problems, but rather that they can play a very significant part in such problems, and must be considered. Unfortunately, such sensitivities are rarely considered, although in my experience they often turn out to be the most important factor affecting behaviour.

# Possible mechanisms of food/ chemical sensitivity

Until recently most of the evidence to support the effects of food/chemical sensitivities (particularly regarding psychological symptoms) has been anecdotal, circumstantial and scientifically limited.

However, over the last few years there has been an emerging body of evidence from many newer scientific disciplines (psychoneuropharmacology, biochemistry and immunology) to make theorising on scientific evidence possible. Presently a number of mechanisms have been proposed through which food/chemical sensitivity may occur. Recent research indicates that the mechanism of food/chemical sensitivity probably involves *functional* as opposed to *organic* disturbances in a number of systems within the body including the immune system, the endogenous opiate system (EOS), the liver, neurotransmitter metabolism in the central nervous system (CNS) and the blood-brain-barrier (BBB).

Chemical exposure is normally discussed in terms of its toxic effects on the body, that is, when chemicals cause actual tissue damage. But in chemical sensitivity we are referring to much lower levels of chemical exposure, which appear to cause changes in the *way* various systems of the body work together. The various systems in the body mesh together like a set of gears—each gear (system) depending on the other gears (systems) to run smoothly. When chemical exposure is at toxic levels, the gears actually break causing damage to other gears as well. But at low levels of chemical exposure the gears may simply lose a few teeth causing a grinding of other gears and problems in the *way* they work together. As gears with missing teeth cannot mesh properly, so systems within the body cannot interact smoothly if there is dysfunction in any one system.

## The Blood-Brain-Barrier (BBB)

As the central nervous system (CNS) cannot store the micronutrients it needs, the BBB's function is to control carefully which substances are allowed into the CNS; in which quantities and at which times. Changes in these functions of the BBB cause dramatic changes in the metabolism of neurotransmitters within the CNS, and therefore cause fluctuating changes in behaviour and mood. (Neurotransmitters are the chemical messengers allowing nerve cells to communicate with each other).

Some factors known to affect BBB functioning are:

(1) Kinins (immune complexes formed in response to an allergic reaction) can circulate to the BBB via the circulatory system, and are known to attack the BBB and to affect its functioning.

(2) Toxic substances can attack and pass through the BBB and affect the CNS. For example, mercury and aluminium may particularly effect the CNS when there is a chronic calcium and magnesium deficiency. Pesticides and herbicides also appear to affect the BBB as well as the CNS.

(3) Food additives, for example erthrosine, can alter the function of the BBB.

(4) The composition of meals can affect BBB functioning. For instance, it is now known that the composition of meals eaten by normal (non-sensitive) people can effect the transport of food micronutrients across the BBB, and hence effect the metabolism of neurotransmitters such as serotonin and dopamine. Both of these neurotransmitters are likely to be involved in food/chemical sensitivity. In fact, amino acids found in food and needed to make such neurotransmitters are presently being prescribed to help sleep and depressive disorders (eg: Tryptophan is an amino-acid found in milk and is needed by the CNS to make serotonin which is an important neurotransmitter involved in sleep and mood). Changing

the composition of a meal (eg: the ratio of carbohydrate to protein) can produce psychological changes large enough to show up clearly with psychological testing.

This has important implications when testing patients for sensitivities. Test meals consist of two to three times a normal size serving of the food. If the test meal is a carbohydrate food eaten at lunchtime, then resulting psychological symptoms may be due to a *perfectly normal* response to an increase in the amount of tryptophan available to make serotonin in the brain rather than a sensitivity reaction.

The case of vitamin B12 is an example of how the effects of a substance permeating the BBB may influence behaviour. It has been known for some time that B12 is particularly useful in treating depression, senility and mood swings in Vietnam war veterans exposed to pesticides and herbicides. I have also found B12 useful for food/chemical sensitive patients with psychological symptoms.

Research on many depressed and senile patients has shown that while blood cell levels of vitamin B12 may be normal or high, the B12 levels in the CNS may be extremely low. This suggests some sort of BBB malfunction is inhibiting B12 transport into the CNS.

In patients who respond to vitamin B12 and other dietary supplements, it may well be that their sensitivities cause malfunctioning of the BBB, necessitating much higher levels of B12 than normal to be in the bloodstream in order for enough to get through the BBB and become available to the CNS.

(5) The BBB undergoes functional changes with development. If food/chemical sensititivies are affecting the BBB in a developing child, they may well affect the maturing of the BBB. This would have a dramatic effect on CNS development and behaviour.

(6) Disturbances in functioning of the BBB and in the availability of nutrients *in the right form* to cross through the BBB owing to changes in liver function. These

changes in liver function can result from prolonged emotional stress, exposure to chemicals and certain types of medication.

The role of the liver in behaviour is only just starting to be explored. Up to now all attention has perhaps understandably been focused on the brain. (Although one must remember that even Hippocrates discussed 'black bile' from the liver and its effect on mood).

Dr Cees Van Tiggelen has formulated theories on this role of the liver based on his own research and wide literature surveys.

His new theory on the possible role of the liver is consistent with my own clinical observations that many chemical and food sensitivity patients respond extraordinarily well to supplementation to improve liver function (and also in general with amino acids, trace minerals—particularly chromium, zinc, magnesium, calcium and iodine—and vitamins B12 and B1).

Dr Van Tiggelen and others have suggested that altered liver function can mean the liver cannot convert these minerals, vitamins and amino acids into the right form to be used by the brain and the immune system.

Dr Van Tiggelen has pointed out the strong similarities between hibernation in animals in which inescapable stress (in this case climatic conditions) induces liver changes which effectively cut off vital nutrients to the brain and immune system so that the body 'shuts off' or goes to sleep until the stress is removed with the return of better weather in spring, and depression in humans. From my own clinical experience I have often been struck by the apparent 'safety valve' nature of many people's depression as a reaction to physical and/or emotional stress they are powerless to control.

In other words, the depression may actually be a very necessary time out period in a person's life and may be the body's way of avoiding physical consequences of uncontrollable stress.

However, once this 'hibernation' starts in humans as a

result of the changes in liver function it can be very difficult to 'turn it off' as, unlike in animals, it is not as a rule tied to changes in the seasons.

By giving patients appropriate supplements, Dr Van Tiggelen and I have both found clinically that you can apparently overcome the liver-induced deficiencies in the brain and immune system and trigger a 'waking up' of the person and, apparently, a restoring of normal liver function.

This has exciting possibilities for the future not only for psychological problems but also for children with learning difficulties, memory problems and so called 'attention deficit disorder' as these children appear to have altered liver function which prevents the availability of crucial nutrients for the development of their central nervous systems.

By prescribing supplements and removing physical stressors (such as sensitivities and chemical exposures) and emotional stressors, appropriate liver function can be restored and the availability of these nutrients to the brain improved.

It must be realised that if a baby is exposed to chemicals and certain kinds of medication given to the mother during pregnancy (eg: cigarette smoke, alcohol, industrial chemicals, pesticides and herbicides, antihypertensives) then these changes in liver function can cause decreased availability of nutrients in the crucial period of development before the baby is even born.

## Pharmacological effects of food/ chemical sensitivity

Many substances naturally occurring in foods can mimic the molecular structure of neurotransmitters, and hence cause behavioural changes in sensitive people. Amines are the most common of such substances, some being structurally similar to hormones within the body, and are usually either psychoactive (acting on the CNS) or vasoactive (acting on the blood vessels). Tyramine, dopamine, histamine and serotonin are all examples of biologically active amines.

For instance, the chemical messenger, or neurotransmitter, serotonin appears to regulate carbohydrate cravings and has been implicated as playing a role in migraine headaches, sleep patterns, aggression in children and some types of depression. In the brain serotonin is manufactured from the dietary amino acid Tryptophan; however, serotonin is also present in many fruits and vegetables, especially bananas.

Although it is important to have an awareness of the many pharmacological reactions which can occur after the consumption/digestion of foods containing naturally occurring toxins or substances which structurally resemble neurotransmitters, it is equally important to realise that only certain sensitive individuals get emotional and/or physical symptoms from the ingestion of these substances.

## The endogenous opiate system

The endogenous opiate system (EOS) of the body is one of the most exciting discoveries in recent years, and is likely to prove the link which explains the connection between the immune system and the central nervous system.

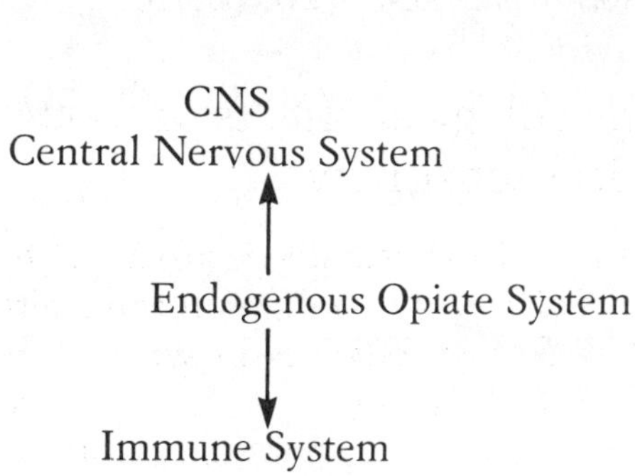

It is thought that incomplete digestion of proteins in the digestive system may form opiate-like substances which could pass through the gut wall into the bloodstream and circulate to the brain. In the brain these 'opiate imitators' could trigger inappropriate responses by the central nervous system.

The endogenous opiate system appears to regulate our reactions to the environment around us, and particularly to stress. The EOS has a pleasure–reward function (eg: it is involved in the 'high' feeling we get when something unbelievably good happens to us), and also acts to control pain and modulate food and water intake. The EOS completes these functions by releasing what is known as endogenous opiates, which are naturally occurring substances in the body similar in chemical structure to morphine. There are two types of endogenous opiates–enkephalins and endorphins.

There is now sufficient evidence to suggest that endorphins and enkephalins actively regulate the immune response, and also that they act as mediators via the circulatory system between the CNS and the immune system. Hence any upset in the functioning of the EOS could effect both the immune system and neurotransmitters within the CNS, and therefore cause psychological symptoms. In fact, there is some evidence to show that the immune cells of sensitive patients will produce opiates when exposed to an allergen, which strongly suggests the EOS is involved in the mechanism of food/chemical sensitivity.

In particular, it appears that the EOS may modulate the dopamine and noradrenaline neurotransmitter systems. Indeed, many of the psychological and physiological symptoms due to food/chemical sensitivity are consistent with a malfunction of these neurotransmitters' metabolism, for instance panic attacks, hallucinations and depression.

## A possible role of Dopamine

Dopamine, a biologically active amine, is a neurotransmitter within the brain. Patients with Parkinson's disease have insufficient dopamine within their CNS. A feature of this illness is very jerky rather than smooth eye movements, and other visual problems, due to a lack of dopamine available to the dopamine receptors in the retina and to the muscles controlling eye movement.

In testing patients for chemical sensitivity I have sometimes found a marked change in the smoothness of eye tracking. Patients' eye movements (particularly children) can become extremely jerky and their eyes lose the ability to coordinate together smoothly. This may suggest that when some patients are reacting to a particular substance, it causes a decrease in the availability of dopamine to their eyes' dopamine receptors.

In the next chapter we look at which behaviour problems are associated with sensitivity.

CHAPTER TWO

# *Behaviour Problems and Sensitivity*

Apart from physical symptoms, food/chemical sensitivities are most likely to produce problems in mood (particularly aggression, anxiety and depression), level of arousal (hyperactivity, overactivity, hypoactivity), sleep (insomnia, nightmares, night terrors etc.), eating patterns (anorexia or binge eating), coordination and learning.

A range of secondary psychological problems can develop as a result of these primary problems and these will be discussed in Part Two.

## Behaviour problems often associated with sensitivities

### Primary problems

Level of arousal—disturbances can lead to:

- Hyperactivity
- Hypoactivity
- Lethargy/chronic fatigue
- Anxiety, phobias, panic attacks

Sleep disturbances
- Insomnia
- Disturbed, restless sleep
- Nightmares
- Night terrors

Mood changes (Often described as having a 'Jeckyl and Hyde' personality)
- Euphoria
- Depression/flat mood
- Aggression

Eating disorders
- Anorexia
- Binge eating

Weight
- Obesity
- Underweight

Toilet training problems
- Bedwetting
- Soiling
- Frequency

## Secondary problems

- Intelligence
- Social skills—social isolation
  - —social rejection
- Frustration/tantrums
- Inconsequential behaviour
- Learning difficulties

## Level of arousal

People with sensitivities often report feelings and exhibit behaviour characteristic of being 'spaced out', extremely lethargic, or 'hyped up'.

To carry out normal daily activities the brain must regulate our level of alertness in the same way that a dimmer switch can regulate the amount of light. If we are too alert we burn up unnecessary energy constantly being 'on guard' for possible physical or emotional attack. This leads to anxiety and fatigue. If we are not alert enough then we cannot respond adequately to physical or psychological demands. The brain must set our 'dimmer' (our level of arousal) to an appropriate setting for the demands on us at the time, then change the setting as our circumstances change.

With sensitivity patients it appears that this 'dimmer' in their brains can be triggered by foods/chemicals and cause changes which are inappropriate to the demands of the situation, eg: falling asleep while driving. These changes in arousal can be anywhere between sleep, underarousal (hypoactive) and overarousal (overactive/hyperactive).

Overactivity or hyperactivity is more commonly reported in children. These children are demanding and highly disruptive in class. They can't keep still and are exhausting not just for adults but for their peers as well. Their inconsequential behaviour—behaviour indicating a negligible concept of past mistakes or future consequences—makes them unpredictable and erratic and extremely difficult to discipline. They tend to live for the minute. Because they are so demanding they are highly visible and can become scapegoats at school and in the family. This type of child has his or her 'dimmer' turned up full!

When you try and explain something to such a child (or adult!) they may look at your blankly. It doesn't matter how many times or how simply you explain something, they seem perpetually confused.

Their attention span is usually very short and the adults often say they can read the same page in a book ten times and still not be able to take it in.

Other consequences of inappropriate arousal can be major problems with concentration and memory—particularly auditory memory. Patients often complain of feeling confused and out of touch with what's going on—'like functioning in a fog'. They often appear dazed and the lethargy they feel can be overwhelming. One patient described it to be 'like climbing Mt Everest with a lead coat on'.

Visual memory does not appear to be affected as much as auditory memory but this may be a cultural artifact. We tend to teach visually rather than aurally, so that when memory is impaired the patient may compensate more easily with visual material than aural material.

These patients, particularly children, have difficulty remembering to do more than one thing at a time. For example, if you tell your child to put her lunchbox on the sink, put her school bag away and then she can watch television—she will remember only one item, usually the first or last. She may remember 'go and watch television' because it was the last thing you said and because it provides greater motivation to remember!

Teachers tend to find these children cannot cope with more than one instruction at a time or they start a task and then literally forget what they are doing.

Our testing of these patients shows problems with spontaneous recall rather than recognition, that is, they can take the information in and process it into long-term memory, but they can't recall it at will. Patients often complain of 'knowing it's in my head but I can't get at it'.

The memory problems can also dramatically affect the comprehension of written material. People with these problems tend to read mechanically but have difficulty making sense of the material because they forget the first words of a sentence before they have reached the end of it.

Both adults and children with these problems can be extremely frustrating to teach or work with, particularly as their performance varies. Sometimes they can do what is required easily and efficiently; at other times their performance is disastrous. The erratic nature of their performance means they are often labelled lazy and/or attention-seeking. This misdiagnosis of their behaviour can have appalling consequences. Professionals and parents tend to become increasingly frustrated as all traditional approaches for dealing with such behaviour fail. They feel the child is 'playing on them'. The child is then treated very unsympathetically and often no attempt is made by adults to conceal their contempt of the child from the child.

## Sleep disorders

Sensitivities can cause disturbed restless sleep, insomnia, oversleeping with a 'hangover' feeling in the mornings, nightmares, night terrors and sleep walking.

Parents often say their children's bed sheets 'look like they've been in a spin drier' by the morning as their sleep is so restless. They may also wake feeling as if they have been 'drugged'.

During the night all of us experience cycles of sleep from very light sleep called REM (Rapid Eye Movement) to very deep sleep. Dreams and nightmares are thought to occur in REM sleep. Night terrors are thought to occur in very deep sleep. With nightmares, the child can usually be woken and comforted fairly easily and has some recollection in the morning. Parents who have had a child suffering night terrors know how terrifying they can be for the child (and the parent!). The child starts screaming hysterically, may pull at her skin and night clothes as she visually hallucinates snakes, spiders etc.

crawling over her body. She may also suffer auditory hallucinations and tear at her ears or cover them. The child appears awake as her eyes are open, but is actually deeply asleep. She is unaware of her parents and may physically attack them in a frenzy. These episodes may last ten to thirty minutes, either once or several times a night. In the morning the child usually has no recollection of the night terror, may be pale and lethargic and difficult to wake.

When night terrors occur there is little that can be done. Turning on the lights and the television can provide other visual and auditory stimulation and may reassure the child until she settles. Sometimes, if the terrors occur several times a night, the child will need sedating for the sake of other terrified children in the family and exhausted parents.

One ten-year-old girl called Toni who was brought to me had a very sad history of extremely aggressive outbursts (including throwing furniture, and hospitalising a younger sibling after attacking him). She suffered repeated night terrors every night. She had been diagnosed as psychotic and it had been further recommended that the mother make her daughter a ward of the state. Her behaviour was controlled by large doses of medication.

Within three days of starting an elimination diet she had no more night terrors. By the end of the week Toni was having no aggressive outbursts and no longer needed medication.

## Mood symptoms

Teachers and families of patients often describe the patient as a 'Jeckyl and Hyde' with totally different personalities which can alter, 'like throwing a switch', with no apparent emotional cause.

These unpredictable changes in mood tend to leave teachers, families and peers quite bewildered. They feel at a loss as to how to respond, since they often 'sense' that the patient can't control him or herself. The most common mood symptoms involve anxiety and panic attacks, depression or a general flatness and 'blunting' of emotional responsiveness, and unprovoked aggression which can be severe and dangerous.

## Coordination problems

These can be either fine motor (eg: poor handwriting) or gross motor problems. Patients whose sensitivities affect the coordination tend to be clumsy, bump into things and have a poor sense of where the body begins and ends in space. Intensive perceptual motor programmes can help these children but the degree of coordination still tends to vary with exposure to an allergen.

## Hallucinations

This is a rare sensitivity reaction but it can occur in children and adults. In my experience, visual hallucinations tend to occur more than auditory hallucinations and are more likely to occur at night.

## Eating disorders and weight maintenance

Despite a variety of diets, behaviour modification programmes, exercise programmes etc., many patients find that food/chemical sensitivities are the main cause of eating disorders or their difficulties in maintaining a satisfactory weight.

In these patients, sensitivities appear to cause major disturbances in the area of the brain involved in hunger, satiation, and with metabolic rate. This is consistent with the possible role of the endogenous opiate system in regulating hunger and satiation.

Small amounts of administered opiates tend to stimulate appetite whereas large amounts tend to diminish appetite.

When sensitive to a particular food it seems that this triggers the production of a small amount of opiate which travels via the bloodstream to opiate centres in the brain causing a pleasant sensation. As the effect of this dose wears off, the patient seeks out the food to retrigger the pleasureable opiate response. Hence he or she becomes 'addicted' to the very food to which he or she is sensitive. When patients stop eating that food, they experience a physical 'withdrawal', with symptoms milder but similar to those of withdrawing heroin (an opiate) addicts.

## Toileting problems

It is common for children (and sometimes adults) with sensitivities to have difficulties with bladder and bowel control.

## Bedwetting

If the child appears to 'flood' the bed when he or she wets either once or several times a night it is often best to try the 'bell and alarm' system. With this system, the child lies on a pad which, if wet, will complete an electrical circuit and ring an alarm to wake the child. This can very quickly 'teach' the child to respond to signals in his or her bladder while he or she is asleep.

The child who appears to wet the bed continuously through the night as if his or her bladder was 'leaking' is usually the child with a sensitivity problem and no amount of alarms, behaviour modification, praise or punishment will help until the sensitivity is diagnosed. These children often have an intermittent problem with dry spells and wet spells. Sensitivities can also cause extremely deep sleep ('like she's been drugged') making the alarm system inappropriate as the child does not wake when the bell rings.

## Frequency

Children with sensitivities often suffer from frequency during the day regardless of how much they drink and may get little warning that they need to void resulting in embarassing accidents. This problem is less common in adults.

## Soiling

When diagnosing a child with soiling problems it is extremely important to make a distinction between the child who appears to get little warning that he or she needs to use his or her bowels (peristaltic rushes) and the child who is soiling with well formed normal stools.

A child experiencing peristaltic rushes often doesn't make the toilet. He or she can become extremely upset or do his or her best to hide evidence of the accident from peers and adults (missing undies!). This type of soiling is often characterised by soiled underwear with a very offensive odour but no solid motion. It can be the result of a chronic constipation problem which causes a 'ballooning' of the bowel so that it cannot work smoothly or efficiently. Parents often mistakenly think that the staining of underwear is due to diarrhoea.

This type of problem is best treated by a combination of a sympathetic GP or gastroenterologist to manage the constipation and get the bowel working properly, and systematic diagnosis and treatment for sensitivity. It is likely that sensitivities caused the constipation in the first place. If adequate investigation of the sensitivities is not pursued, the problem will probably recur.

The child soiling with normal solid motions is best treated by a psychologist looking at psychological factors which would account for the behaviour.

# Secondary problems

## Intelligence

Intelligence is a general term used to describe the ability of an individual to adapt to and manipulate his or her environment to fulfill his or her physical and psychological needs.

To act intelligently, an individual must perceive his or her environment accurately in order to respond appropriately.

The effects that sensitivities can have on level of arousal, mood and short-term memory can make accurate perception of the physical and emotional environment impossible. Over time, these patients' view of their world can become grossly distorted making their responses to the environment often illogical and inappropriate.

Their 'intelligence' is affected as they cannot adapt to or manipulate effectively an environment which they do not perceive accurately.

The consequences of this and the primary symptoms, particularly if not diagnosed properly, can lead to secondary problems. These will be dealt with in Part Two.

Highly intelligent children and adults often unconsciously develop strategies to overcome the effects of their sensitivities on intellectual functioning. These patients are often perceived by others as coping quite normally, whereas in fact their true ability level is being masked.

Of course, all these symptoms can also be produced by factors other than food sensitivities. In the next chapter we look at how to determine whether these symptoms are likely to be predominantly sensitivity-related, or are caused by some other factor.

# *CHAPTER THREE*

# *Diagnosing Behaviour Problems*

To decide whether a person's psychological symptoms are likely to be sensitivity-related, the following features must be considered.

1. Family history
2. Patient's history
3. 'Trigger events'
4. Presence of physical *and* psychological symptoms
5. Relative importance of other factors in the ecological model of behaviour

## 1. Family history

If there is a strong family history of traditional allergy (asthma, eczema, hayfever) then it is more likely that sensitivities could be causing psychological symptoms. However, if there is no family history of traditional allergies it is still possible that sensitivities could be involved, particularly if there is a significant personal physical history.

# 2. Patient's physical history

Patients who have sensitivities typically have a childhood or current history of many of the following physical symptoms which can be allergy or sensitivity related. They may report that with time their symptoms have tended to change, eg: eczema → asthma → hayfever → migraine.

## Significant symptoms:

Mother suffering prolonged morning sickness during pregnancy

Adverse reactions to immunisations and drugs

Absence of breastfeeding

**Digestive system**

Colic

Vomiting

Baby refusing breastfeeding

Diarrhoea and/or constipation

Soiling, particularly if offensive odour

Flatulence or bloating

Nausea

**Urinary system**

Vaginitis (particularly at night), non specific urethritis

Bedwetting, frequency

Cystitis

**Respiratory system**

Asthma, persistent cough

Repeated chest infections, bronchitis or croup

Hayfever, runny nose, sinusitis

Sore throats or hoarseness

Repeated ear infections and/or hearing loss

**Circulatory system**

Blood noses

Pallor, dark circles under eyes

Night sweats

Sensitive to cold or heat

Palpitations

**Musclo-skeletal**

Arthralgia (aching joints, 'growing pains')

Myalgia (aching muscles particularly legs) stiff neck and shoulders

Arthritis (particularly rheumatoid)

**Central nervous system**

Irritability

Blurred vision

Headaches and migraine

Epilepsy

Unexplained high temperatures

Behavioural symptoms (as mentioned previously)

**Endrocrine system**

Premenstrual syndrome

Adverse reactions to the pill or other hormone therapy

**Immune system**

Auto-immune diseases

**Trauma**

Major accidents involving physical injury

## 3. 'Trigger' event

Patient may say that symptoms were 'triggered' by a certain event:

**Emotional traumas**
- bereavement
- change of job
- separation
- car accidents, etc.
- prolonged emotional stress

**Physical traumas**
- exposure to toxic chemicals
- flu or viral illness, particularly glandular fever
- major injury
- thyroid problems
- pregnancy
- severe allergic reaction, eg: to a drug or an insect bite
- nutritional deficiencies

## 4. Presence of physical and psychological symptoms

*The most important clue to sensitivities being a significant factor in a psychological symptom is the presence of physical AND psychological symptoms together.*

It is possible but highly unlikely that a psychological problem would have a significant sensitivity component if there are no physical symptoms.

Often patients are used to a multitude of relatively minor problems in their physical functioning and accept these physical symptoms as 'just me'. They gave up mentioning them to health professionals years ago and have suffered in silence.

It is therefore very important that health professionals suspecting sensitivity ask specifically if certain symptoms occur.

# 5. Relative importance of other factors

To finalise the diagnosis it is necessary to consider and appropriately weight all the other factors operating for a particular patient within the ecological model.

This can be best explained by looking at case histories.

## Case history 1: 'Steve'

Vietnam War veteran, age thirty-nine

**Presenting symptoms**
The following symptoms had been present in varying degrees and duration since his service in Vietnam:

hallucinations, irritability, chronic nervous exhaustion, morbid fears, depression, anxiety attacks, insomnia and nightmares, unreasonable anger and aggressive outbursts, difficulty concentrating, poor memory, cold hands and feet, headaches, skin rashes, blurred vision, digestive upsets, hot flushes and blackouts.

**Medication at time of referral**
(There had been a great variation in amounts of medication over the years.)

Euhypnos, 20 mg at night; Sinequan, 50 mg at night; Ducene, 5 mg twice daily.

**Past treatment**
Multiple psychiatric hospital admissions; years of regular psychiatric treatment including heavy medication.

**Diagnosis using the ecological model**
**Physical internal factors:**

chronic back pain from war injury; psychological symptoms relieved by medication suggesting a physical basis; *Functional Hypoglycaemia (symptom score 110); mineral imbalance—high toxic mineral levels, high copper, low calcium, magnesium levels.

**Physical external factors:**

Melathion exposure (In Vietnam: tents and bedding were sprayed and it was even in drinking water); multiple exposures to defoliants; symptoms now 'triggered' by certain situations, eg: mowing lawn, driving long distances.

**Emotional**

Self —war neurosis, guilt.

Family —extremely supportive wife; problems with relationships with extended family members.

Community—as a Vietnam veteran ostracised and felt many of his needs were ignored by Veteran's Affairs.

**Treatment using model**

Supportive counselling (basically RET); diet; supplements; diagnosis and management of food/chemical sensitivities.

---

* *Functional Hypoglycaemia: not to be confused with very rare True Hypoglycaemia where blood glucose levels are chronically low. Functional Hypoglycaemia is a common condition in sensitivity patients which can be diagnosed from a six-hour Glucose Tolerance Test (GTT). The body has trouble maintaining satisfactory levels of blood glucose appropriate to the body's needs at the time, ie: it is either too high or too low or rising and falling too rapidly.*

Progress after a few months:

**Medication**

Down to 1 Euhypnos at night

**Physical symptoms**

Blackouts stopped; rashes much better; energy increased; chronic nervous exhaustion gone; very few nightmares; insomnia gone; symptom score down to 65 (Functional Hypoglycaemia).

**Psychological symptoms**

Hallucinations stopped; mood lability decreased; depression—episodic only; increased ability to handle interpersonal relationships; irritability decreased.

**Prognosis**

Needs occasional supportive counselling and supplements. Must keep to diet and supplements.

This case history of a Vietnam veteran is particularly interesting as it illustrates the problems of toxicity versus sensitivity. The claims of Vietnam veterans that exposure to pesticides and herbicides has caused damage to their physical and emotional health have been well publicised.

Apart from the obvious political reluctance to acknowledge any such connection, there has also been the problem that many of the veterans' claims have related to functional rather than organic complaints (apart from the claims of birth defects in their children as a result of their own exposure to chemicals in Vietnam).

Rather than look at Vietnam veterans in terms of toxic damage (although I have no doubt that this has also occurred), in clinical practice I was immediately struck by the similarity in symptoms between these men and my sensitivity patients.

Once I looked at their problems in terms of sensitivity, particularly to chemicals, their symptoms made much more sense. The symptoms could then be very effectively managed after careful diagnosis of these sensitivities and treatment with supplements, diet and minimising chemical exposure.

When one investigates the living and working environments of sensitivity patients, there is often a history of very significant chemical exposure from pesticide spraying in and around the home. I strongly suspect that in many ways sensitivities are the first signs of toxic exposures. This is consistent with the current view of neuropsychotoxicology, which is that behavioural changes are likely to be observed well before physical changes as a person strives to maintain homeostasis within his or her body. Hence functional changes will occur in the way systems are working together before physical damage occurs.

## Case history 2: 'Jo-anne'

Thirteen-year-old girl

**Presenting symptoms**

Obesity; binge eating (particularly sugar); chronic fatigue; concentration and memory impaired; headaches; serious depression.

**Diagnosis of GP**

Depressed and obese because 'eating like a greedy pig'.

**Previous treatment**

Anti-depressants; counselling from very experienced counsellor.

**Diagnosis using the ecological model**

**Physical internal factors**

Genetic — strong history of obesity and thyroid problems in family

Nutritional — dietary history revealed very poor diet. Physical symptoms (bleached nails, sleep disturbance, cravings) suggested nutritional imbalance, particularly regarding chromium and zinc.

Psychological—depression relieved a little by anti-depressants

**Physical external factors**

Most weight gain and binging since moving to a house with gas heating and recently painted throughout. Binging always worse in winter. Mould in bedroom behind curtains and on floor of cupboard.

**Emotional factors**

Self —low self esteem, withdrawn, unresolved grief for father's death, socially isolated.

Family —dramatic change in financial status since father's death; move from family farm in small community to inner Melbourne suburb; mother working very hard so much less time with children.

School —Move from very small rural school to large multicultural suburban school.

Community—move from close-knit, supportive local community to anonymity of suburbs with little community support.

**Diagnosis and treatment**

When the mother brought her child to see me the child was getting worse not better, despite intensive counselling of the child and her mother, and anti-depressant medication.

The analysis of the factors above illustrate the complexity of her problems. In this case insufficient attention had been given to the physical factors operating.

This young girl was found to have a mild thyroid deficiency which was contributing to her problems. But it was not the whole answer.

She also showed dramatic changes in mood and appetite when tested for mould and gas sensitivity. Dietary manipulation disclosed similar problems with milk, wheat and sugar.

By diagnosing and managing the physical problems her mood improved dramatically and her weight steadily decreased without counting calories. She was then much more able to respond to counselling to resolve her grief and make adjustments to her new life.

These case histories illustrate how vital it is that priorities for more detailed diagnostic testing and treatment strategies be worked out very carefully. Generally speaking, physical problems need to be tackled first. However, the diagnosis and management of significant food/chemical sensitivities can put enormous demands on all the family emotionally and financially.

For this reason the programme must be individualised for a particular patient in the context of his or her family and finances. Often what is technically correct in a textbook sense can be a disaster in practice.

For instance, a woman came to me after being 'processed' by another health professional according to what was technically correct for diagnosing sensitivity. However, she was becoming steadily worse 'for no apparent reason'. A little further discussion revealed that she had been on a merry-go-round of testing and severe elimination diets while her marriage was breaking up, her eldest child was receiving treatment for leukaemia and her youngest had been run over by a car!

It wasn't sensitivities causing her weight loss but severe emotional strain and just not eating. It was extremely difficult obtaining the unusual foods allowed by her diet sitting in hospital waiting rooms!

CHAPTER FOUR

# Methods of Diagnosing and Treating Sensitivities

## What causes sensitivities?

There are many theories on why people develop sensitivities but as yet there is still very little research to support them.

The body's immune system appears to work like an early warning radar system, telling the body what's happening in the external environment and relaying this information to the central nervous system (CNS) and other areas of the body so that appropriate responses can be made.

It is known that increasing chemical exposure, particularly of herbicides and pesticides, does 'weaken' the immune system and make it less able to cope with environmental assault or to maintain proper immune vigilance within the body itself.

Much has been written about whether the growth of candida (a yeast which normally grows in the bowel) is the main culprit in food sensitivity. There is no doubt that many patients improve on an anti-candida diet and supplements but whether that is due to the growth of candida being impeded or some other factor, it is extremely difficult to tell. Not all patients respond to an anti-candida 'regime'. Perhaps those that do, improve because they have eliminated foods to which they are actually sensitive. Of course the patient doesn't really mind what the reason is if he or she feels much better! It may be that environmental chemicals have weakened the bowel's immune system, thus allowing an overgrowth of candida.

For patients with multiple sensitivities an anti-candida regime may make things worse by unnecessarily limiting their diet.

In the absence of hard scientific evidence, the clinical evidence suggests to me that sensitivities are a subtle sign that the immune system is under siege from an increasingly chemical world.

# Diagnosis of allergies and sensitivities

## Concurrent diagnosis

Once it has been established that food/chemical sensitivity is likely to be a significant factor, accurate diagnosis is crucial. Ideally all sensitivities, ie: inhalant, food, chemical or contact, need to be diagnosed concurrently as each sensitivity can affect the severity of others. For example, if a predominantly chemical problem is minimised this can improve food sensitivity: removing milk from the diet of a milk-sensitive person can improve that person's hayfever.

In fact, traditional allergists and clinical ecologists (health professionals dealing with environmental sensitivities) tend to think in terms of the total allergic and sensitivity 'load' of a patient. Patients can often adapt their physiology to a large number of sensitivities or allergies without significant symptoms. But then a 'trigger event' which stresses the whole immune system or exposure to a large amount of a particular allergen which overloads the system can cause symptoms to develop. (An allergen is a substance which can cause allergy or sensitivity in a particular individual. A substance may be an allergen to one person and not to another.)

One patient could eat chocolate with no ill effects until exam time. As the stress of exams was added to the load on his immune system the total load on his body became too much and he developed severe migraine if he ate chocolate. Once exams were over he could eat chocolate again without symptoms.

## Diagnosis of inhalant allergies/sensitivities

Inhalant allergies/sensitivities refers to reactions caused by naturally occurring airborne particles (dust mite, grass pollens, moulds etc.). These reactions can be traditional Type 1 allergy where a substance in the blood called IGe (Immunoglobulin type E) reacts with an antigen to produce histamine. The symptoms tend to be asthma, hayfever, rashes. The moulds can also cause behavioural symptoms (particularly mood change, level of arousal, sleep disturbance, hallucinations) and these reactions are probably non-IgE mediated. Inhalent allergies causing traditional Type 1 symptoms can be fairly accurately diagnosed using either 'prick' tests or intradermal skin tests. Inhalent sensitivities causing non-Type 1 symptoms, eg: hallucinations from moulds, must be diagnosed using other techniques.

## Diagnosis of allergies/sensitivities which cause behavioural and psychological symptoms

There are a large number of tests used to diagnose the various types of allergy. Unfortunately, many of these tests can give misleading results when looking at the broader problem of sensitivity reaction rather than just traditional allergy.

Traditional allergists use mainly skin (prick tests, intradermal tests) and blood tests. These tests are inadequate and unreliable for testing the reactions that cause psychological performance and behavioural symptoms.

All tests currently being used for diagnosing allergy and sensitivity reactions which cause physical or behavioural problems have severe limitations and can be most unreliable unless careful attention is given to how they are carried out and under what conditions. The only tests discussed here are those which I have found to be reliable clinically for diagnosing behavioural and psychological symptoms.

Patients with significant sensitivities (particularly chemical) cannot afford to waste time and money on unreliable testing. If not properly diagnosed their illness can deteriorate to the point where it is impossible for them to recover or resume work.

Patients with minor problems often find 'alternative' diagnostic techniques satisfactory, as only relatively minor dietary restrictions are recommended. However, before spending a lot of money on testing it should be remembered that a good patient and dietary history is sufficient to indicate the six most important food sensitivities.

**Allergen** — a substance which can cause a allergy or sensitvity in a particular person.

**Allergen Extract** — these are made by disolving a measured amount of allergen in liquid. Different dilutions of extracts are made to give different strength extracts. One way of making dilutions is as follows:
No. 1 dilution is one part allergen to ten parts diluent.
No. 2 dilution is one part allergen to one hundred parts diluent.
No. 3 dilution is one part allergen to one thousand parts diluent.
And so on, usually up to No. 10.

## Types of tests

### 1. Skin tests

These tests involve placing drops of allergen extracts (eg: dust mite) on the skin and then pricking the skin to see if the extract causes a lump or weal to develop. The degree of sensitivity can be gauged by the size of the weal using different dilutions of extract.

As the skin tests are testing for IgE mediated allergy, and as some inhalents appear to cause non IgE sensitivity reactions, sublingual drop testing should also be done when considering psychological symptoms.

### 2. Sublingual drop testing

This method involves placing a particular strength of allergen extract (usually No. 1, the strongest) under the tongue where there is very rapid absorption into the bloodstream and seeing if objective and subjective symptoms develop. This type of testing is most useful for testing chemicals and moulds.

As patients can often taste the drops and there is a large degree of subjective reporting by patients, it is essential for people (particularly children) reporting behavioural symptoms that this type of testing is done in conjunction with psychological assessment.

Psychological assessment can control for other factors (eg: expectation effects) which can influence results. The psychological testing done as part of psychological assessment can often detect reactions of which the patient is unaware (eg: memory changes, concentration difficulties, coordination). This is particularly important when testing children as unreliable or inaccurate test results can have profound consequences for their social and emotional development and educational achievement. For patients making medico-legal claims (*even when the symptoms are predominantly physical*), sublingual testing must be carried out in conjunction with psychological assessment, to determine whether psychological factors may be causing the symptoms. Otherwise the credibility of the results can be seriously challenged.

Repeated sublingual drop testing increases the likelihood of psychological factors, such as the patient's expectations, affecting the reliability of test results. Also, in many clinics and in hospital testing patients can 'learn' symptoms (both physical and psychological) from observing others being tested. 'Learned' immune responses have even been observed in animals. For this reason I have found it more useful to test for two or three of the most likely chemical offenders based on an environmental history. If the results are positive then the overall chemical exposure in the home and the workplace should be minimised. Testing must be carried out so that patients cannot observe or hear others being tested.

If a person reacts to two or three chemicals then they are a chemically sensitive patient and they are likely to react to other chemicals as well. I have found repeated testing to find long lists of 'passed' or 'failed' chemicals can be unreliable and give patients a wrong impression of their chemical sensitivity. Professionals and patients can get bogged down in details and not see the overall problem of minimising general chemical exposure. For example, one patient successfully eliminated a long list of 'failed' chemicals from her home but continued to wear 'passed' synthetic clothing which she had regularly drycleaned!

Another patient spent a lot of money removing all foam from her furniture. But she continued to run an ironing business from home, exposing herself to the fumes of a multitude of heated synthetics and the residues of a variety of laundry detergents. (She also neglected to change the foam underlay of the ironing board.)

Patients who are chemically sensitive need to minimise *all* chemical exposures at home, work, or school. For example, hanging the newspapers on the clothesline while they 'gas off' (ie: until the smell of the printing has gone) won't help much if you have a leaking gas stove or if you smoke.

### 3. Open tests

These involve actually watching what happens when eating a food or being exposed to a chemical.

#### (i) Food and chemical diaries

These diaries record all the food and drink a patient consumes, under what conditions physically and emotionally, and what symptoms occurred at what time.

As multiple sensitivities tend to mask individual reactions and these reactions can be delayed by days, diaries are rarely a sufficient diagnostic tool in themselves. However, they can be a very useful first step and give a reliable indication of the most likely food and/or chemical sensitivities. A modified elimination diet suggested by interpretation of the diaries can then be tried.

### (ii) Elimination diet

A full elimination diet is based on a detailed dietary history and severely restricts the diet to those foods (sometimes as little as five to eight foods) least likely to cause problems for a particular patient. Elimination diets must be worked out on an individual need basis. The patient stays on this diet for seven days as it takes four to six days for foods to be fully eliminated from the body. By the seventh day the symptoms should have disappeared if all the offending foods were eliminated. Foods are then tested one at a time and reactions noted over the next three to four weeks.

The extreme elimination diet is a full fast for five days consuming only pure filtered water or distilled water but this is rarely done with out-patients.

For patients suffering food/chemical sensitivity, elimination diets are really the only reliable methods of testing foods. Many other methods are undoubtedly easier but sooner or later patients with significant problems have to resort to the elimination diet. Unfortunately, if patients leave this method to 'later' rather than as soon as possible they can be extremely debilitated and their health problems infinitely more complex to work out.

In children particularly, delaying accurate diagnosis can have catastrophic effects emotionally, socially and educationally.

### (iii) Environmental control unit (ECU)

The open tests described above can be difficult to carry out and unreliable if the patient is suffering from multiple chemical sensitivity. If no significant emotional or psychological factors are involved, another way to test such patients is in an environmental control unit (ECU).

An ECU is usually located within a normal hospital. The ECU is sealed off from the rest of the hospital with its own specialised air-conditioning system. No chemicals or plastics are allowed into the ECU. All furniture, bedding, clothing, toiletries and cleaning agents must be derived from natural materials and be as inert as possible. All water is filtered or distilled.

Patients in the ECU undergo a full five-day fast and in this way all foods and chemicals can be eliminated from the body.

As the body eliminates chemicals and foods the patient may experience a 'physical withdrawal' with mild to severe symptoms as the body re-adapts to not having the stress of the allergens. This 'withdrawal' is also experienced out of hospital by patients on elimination diets.

The patient is then tested by re-introducing foods one at a time and when sufficient foods have been passed chemicals are tested, either sublingually or by direct exposure, in special 'booths' with their own air extraction systems.

This whole procedure takes four to six weeks and patients cannot leave the ECU at all during that time. Admission to an ECU is extremely physically and emotionally demanding for patients and their families. The isolation makes patients very vulnerable emotionally.

The ECU can control physical environmental factors extremely well. Unfortunately, however, confinement in an ECU does introduce a multitude of psychological factors which can interfere with testing and dramatically affect reliability. These factors influence not just patients but have complex effects on staff as well. If not adequately controlled, these psychological variables can have long-term effects for the patient physically and emotionally. The limitations of the ECU are especially important when testing children, patients with behavioural symptoms, or patients with medico-legal claims.

The admission of children to an ECU must be especially carefully considered and the timing arranged to minimise interference with school. It is particularly important that children do not miss the first part of the school year as socially this is a crucial time. The child with health problems who misses this part of school can find him or herself socially isolated for the rest of the year.

Because of the psychological factors operating within the ECU, all patients should be assessed by an experienced clinical psychologist (or educational psychologist for children) before admission to the unit. A similarly qualified psychologist should also monitor and review patients during admission. Sometimes, psychological problems can develop as a result of testing and being confined to hospital. This can mean that, for the sake of a particular patient him or herself, and the overall emotional atmosphere within the ECU, testing may need to be suspended or the patient discharged prematurely.

It is important to realise that ECU admission is simply one method of diagnosis and not necessarily the 'best' method or for the 'worst' patients. Patients often mistakenly believe that because ECU admission has been suggested they must be a 'serious case' and they expect to react to everything they will be tested for. These expectations combine with other psychological factors in the ECU and can set the patient up for psychologically induced reactions which can also produce physical symptoms.

Out-patient testing can control for the significant psychological variables but can be difficult if there is multiple chemical sensitivity.

## Conclusion

To avoid the development of secondary psychological symptoms it is imperative that accurate diagnosis of the food/chemical sensitivity is carried out with due regard to all the factors contributing to the symptoms, and with consideration of the consequences to the patient's family as a whole.

In general, inhalent, food, chemical and contact

allergies/sensitivities need to be looked at together to prevent important sensitivities being missed.

Inhalent sensitivities are diagnosed using skin and sublingual tests. Foods are best diagnosed using elimination diets, and chemicals are best diagnosed using sublingual testing in conjunction with psychological testing and assessment.

The methods used to test patients must be carefully considered for each patient at a particular stage of the illness, eg: sometimes ECU admission is totally inappropriate for a particular patient at one time but becomes the best option at another time.

Generally speaking, children and patients with significant psychological symptoms should be tested as out-patients. Patients with medico-legal claims are most reliably assessed as out-patients in conjunction with psychological assessment.

Owing to the enormous cost, time, and psychological factors involved in ECU admission, all patients (including those with mainly physical symptoms) who have been recommended for admission to ECU should get an independent second opinion. In this way any doubts can be alleviated and resolved before admission and the patient and his or her family's attitudes is as positive as possible. This can greatly reduce conflict and the stressful times that may develop during admission.

# Treatment

### Desensitisation

In practice, traditional allergy treatment is restricted to a desensitisation and avoidance of the offending allergen.

Desensitisation involves giving the patient very small amounts of the allergen he or she is allergic to in increasing dosages over a period of months or years. If the treatment is successful, the patient's immune system seems to learn that the substance isn't worth reacting to and stops producing symptoms on exposure.

Many patients report that they tried desensitisation for the traditional allergies but it didn't work. However, if patients tackle all their allergies and sensitivities together, ie: inhalent, food, chemical and contact, then desensitisation is much more effective. As desensitisation involves a series of injections it can be inappropriate for young children and needle phobic adults.

For the patients I see with predominantly psychological and behavioural symptoms, I have found desensitisation to be helpful only for some inhalents and not for foods or chemicals.

**Homeopathic drops**

For many years it has been known, but not understood, that giving some patients a minute dilution of their allergen as sublingual drops can actually mask symptoms of reactions. The appropriate dosage of drops must be worked out for each patient individually.

For instance, if Dilution No. 1 (one-tenth dilution) of petrochemical extract provokes symptoms, then giving Dilution No. 4 (one ten-thousandth dilution) of petrochemical may 'turn-off' the symptoms for that particular patient. By taking the prescribed strength of drops before or after exposure to an allergen, eg: going out in traffic, patients can minimise their symptoms.

These drops do not work for every patient and can be difficult to administer with children. But they are worth a try for chemical sensitivity and some inhalents (eg: moulds, dust mite). I have not found this method reliable or worth the effort for foods.

I suspect that much of the mechanism of sensitivity will not be fully understood until there is a greater understanding of homeopathy in general. Recent research is providing increasing support for homeopathy as an extremely safe method of treatment.

**Avoidance**

Unfortunately, for many people, avoidance is the only treatment option. For this reason it is crucial that food/chemical sensitivities be diagnosed as early as possible before there are major health problems.

For foods, early diagnosis and avoidance for a few days in an infant and for three to six months in an adult can mean that an offending food may be safely reintroduced into the diet without lifetime avoidance.

For chemical sensitivity the situation is more difficult. Total avoidance of chemicals in our modern world is impossible. The best one can do is minimise one's exposure and take sensible precautions. Many people diagnosed as chemically sensitive feel that moving to the country may help. This is not necessarily so, as the widespread use of highly toxic materials in rural areas can make the country more chemically dangerous than the city.

Before contemplating a move out of your home you should seek expert advice, as it is often far more satisfactory to spend money modifying your present home, whose chemical history you know very well, than moving to a home with an unknown chemical history.

I have now spent several years going into people's homes and considering chemical hazards, and what is most striking is that the major problem can turn out to be quite different to those the patient suspected.

The decision to move must be done on an individual basis, taking into account all the emotional and socioeconomic consequences for the patient and for his or her family.

Theoretically, patients following avoidance treatment should develop better chemical tolerance and be less sensitive. In practice this may not occur as much as is hoped—even if some improvement in tolerance does develop and physical symptoms diminish or disappear, the psychological symptoms associated with problems with chemical exposure can be more difficult to help (particularly memory problems).

## Alternative approaches

Once someone has been diagnosed as chemically/food sensitive, the prospect of avoidance can be extremely daunting. People naturally seek out other ways of minimising their symptoms which may be less socially or emotionally demanding.

The techniques I have found to be of most benefit to patients are dietary supplementation with amino acids (particularly for mood and memory problems), minerals, vitamins, lacto bacillus, lacto bifida, lacto bulgaricum, digestive enzymes etc., homeopathy, acupunture, therapeutic massage, hypnosis and subliminal programming, deep relaxation and meditation. Each patient will find out for him or herself what brings the most benefits but, generally speaking, any method which lowers or relieves stress on the mind or body is likely to be helpful.

Dietary supplements can be particularly helpful to people with sensitivities.

It should be remembered that RDA's (recommended daily allowances) for nutrients are based on the amount of a nutrient needed to be consumed each day to avoid the development of obvious physical and extreme psychological symptoms. Unfortunately, as stated earlier, subtle behavioural symptoms are likely to occur a long time before physical symptoms, so these RDA's can be far lower than what is actually needed by a particular individual to avoid behavioural or psychological symptoms.

Also, RDA's are calculated for the mythical 'average' person and people suffering from sensitivities or who are exposed to chemicals at work, school or at home can have much higher nutrient requirements.

It cannot be assumed that a good diet with no junk food is necessarily supplying adequate nutrients when one considers that the vitamin and mineral content of a food can vary dramatically depending on the type of soil it was grown in, the time of year it was grown, the fertilisers used and even what previous crops were grown in the soil. Add to this the changes in nutrient availability due to processing, packaging and storing, and malabsorption problems common in people with sensitivities and one has to wonder if tables of vitamins and minerals in particular foods really mean much in terms of the nutrients you actually consume compared to a person's individual need.

In a desperate attempt to get better many patients self-prescribe supplements which are inappropriate to their condition. They may do no harm but can waste a great deal of money.

If you feel you or particularly your children may need a supplement, don't just buy something off the shelf but seek advice from an appropriately qualified health professional. (Sometimes health food store owners and pharmacists have appropriate qualifications themselves or can refer you to an appropriate professional in your area).

It is extremely rare for patients to find any of these methods very helpful in themselves. These methods must be used in conjunction with some degree of avoidance of the offending foods and/or chemicals.

# *PART TWO*

# *Effects and Consequences of Sensitivity*

CHAPTER FIVE

# Infants, Children and Adolescents

## Infants

Food and chemical sensitivities can affect babies before they are born. Mothers who binge or consume large amounts of particular foods can create sensitivities in their children—the most common being wheat and milk.

Childen born with sensitivities can be irritable and colicky within hours or a few days of birth. Sometimes they have rashes, sleep fitfully, and give new mothers little cause to delight in motherhood. Babies may refuse the breast or vomit after each feed. They are often more sensitive to pain, changes in temperature, light and noise, and their hands and feet may be unusually cold. Sadly, because of the often unrewarding nature of the child–mother relationship, secondary emotional and behavioural problems often develop.

Such babies suffer chronic pain or discomfort which the one person in life they depend on—their mother—is powerless to relieve. The infant's frustration and anger must be acute, as is that of the mother who finds that no matter what she does she cannot help. Walking the floor for hours on end carrying a whining or screaming baby has a devastating effect on self-esteem, as well as being physically and emotionally exhausting. Only someone who has been in this situation (and very few male professionals have) can understand the torment of the mother and child, the frustration and anger that at times feels like an overwhelming external force. Usually such mothers find their feelings for their child oscillating somewhere between overwhelming love and protectiveness (usually when the child is finally asleep!) to intense hatred towards this tiny thing that has robbed them of sleep and self-respect and the respect of family, friends and partner. 'I must be a bad mother' is the guilty reaction of many. Research involving sleep deprivation, or allowing only interrupted sleep, has had to be terminated after only a few weeks because of the serious psychological consequences to the subjects of the experiment. But we expect mothers of such children to cope single handedly with very little sleep or relief for months on end. It is not surprising that child abuse is a common phenomena in families of such children.

The mother with an allergic baby who does not admit to exhaustion, anger, bitterness and a love/hate relationship with her baby is of more concern than those who do. The repression of feelings which are a normal response to a very abnormal situation can lead to an emotional detachment and clinical objectivity which is more harmful for mother and child.

This 'switching off' from the relationship is one of the most tragic consequences for these babies and their mothers. When the eldest child is allergic the mother may look to her younger children for the rewards of motherhood and emotional comfort she was deprived of with the first.

Even if the younger children are also ill, their demands can be more physical, and less emotionally draining than the two to three-year-old coping with sensitivities and the 'terrible two's' normal frustration and anger as well.

Often it is not the illness which causes rejection of these children but the lack of a definitive diagnosis and, consequently, a tendency to blame the parents.

Children with sensitivities can become the scapegoats within their own family and at school. All family crises and problems are blamed in some way on this particular child who quickly sees him or herself as a 'loser', 'hopeless' and worthless. Even professionals, when faced with the dilemma of a very well-adjusted set of parents and siblings, have been known to shrug their shoulders and dismiss the problem child as a difficult personality or 'just born bad'.

The two-year-old stuck at home with mum and younger sibling quickly realises that attention (even if negative) comes through disruptive behaviour. Add these emotional influences to a child who, due to his or her sensitivities, is already impulsive, active and very moody, and one has the potential for a very unhappy child with quite distraught parents. Siblings also learn to use the allergic child to their advantage, taking every opportunity to point out their own 'goodness' and the 'badness' of the sibling.

In my early training as a psychologist very little attention was paid to the effects of physical health on behaviour unless these were relatively gross physical problems, eg: diabetes, birth trauma, genetic defect, meningitis, etc. Behaviour problems were predominately diagnosed and treated by a mixture of counselling and behaviour therapy imposed on the parents, the school and the child. The child was usually seen as the victim whose overt behaviour was the result of various forces beyond his or her control. I had a mental picture of the child as a little cork that had been thrown mid-Atlantic and was powerless in the face of gigantic waves, (namely school and society) and even bigger icebergs—the child's parents.

# Kindergarten and school

Once the child with sensitivities leaves the physical and emotional environment of home his or her poor ability to adapt physically and emotionally make kindergarten and school adjustments even more difficult.

Kindergartens and schools are becoming increasingly physically hazardous, not just for people with sensitivities, but for healthy people as well. In the 'old days', schools had bare hardwood floors, no duplicated material, no heat, wooden furniture, chalk pencils and paper. The most health hazardous items were probably chalk dust and the inkwell and the sharp pen nib of the person sitting behind you!

These days, the average classroom has treated synthetic carpet, gas heaters, no opening windows (owing to the requirements of the heating and/or air-conditioning or to the fact that they were painted over long ago), few, if any, ventilators in the wall, plastic chairs, fresh duplicated material, spirit pens, glues, soft plastic covered books, plastic storage containers, teachers wearing aftershave or perfume, twenty to thirty warm bodies wearing synthetic uniforms (usually polyester mixes) and often synthetic underwear as well. Heating and humidity is highly variable and rarely comfortable.

Also, each person in the room pumps out carbon dioxide into the air and removes oxygen. We are often expecting children to learn in highly polluted air—and this does not include the car exhaust, petrochemicals and airborne pollution often surrounding a suburban school. Add to this large areas of vapourising bitumen in the school ground and you get some idea of the chemical soup to which children are exposed. Schools and modern work environments are producing *pickled people*!

You may be wondering whether these problems, although extremely important to the individual sufferer, are important for the community.

It has been estimated that between twenty-five to sixty percent of the population in Australia suffer from the traditional wheezes and sneezes type allergies. (The estimates of the incidence of traditional allergy vary enormously, depending on which medical authority is speaking. Individual specialists have even given figures of seventy percent.) From my work in schools and in private practice I would estimate that at least thirty percent of people, and probably more, suffer from significant food/chemical sensitivities affecting their psychological performance and emotional behaviour. This means that in the average classroom at least ten children, including those with more obvious traditional allergies, are having their educational achievement and social development affected by the chemicals they breathe and the food they eat.

In the classroom these children are described as either lazy, too active, lethargic, irritable, talkative, easily distracted, naughty, aggressive, noisy, sulky, immature and nuisances. Socially and educationally their responses tend to be inappropriate. They laugh at the wrong time, their coordination is poor. They are erratic in everything they do. Their performance and social skills vary, depending on whether they are being affected by their sensitivities or not.

The areas most affected are coordination (gross and fine motor), concentration, mood and memory (particularly auditory memory).

Because their social behaviour is so unpredictable other children tend to avoid them (as do adults). It is difficult to make close friendships with someone who is even-tempered, pleasant and caring one moment and aggressive, impulsive and destructive the next.

Teachers find these children particularly confusing. Because their performance varies so greatly they are often accused of being stubborn and lazy.

If others find them so confusing, this is nothing to the

anguish experienced by the children themselves. In testing sessions many of these children have told me how frightened they are by their rapid changes in mood, and inability to do their schoolwork. They make bewildered statements about their feelings: 'Sometimes my inside gets all messed up and nothing works properly'; 'Maybe I've got a brain tumor eating my brain'.

Observing sensitive children during reactions to chemical extracts reminds me of my time as a student. In the behavioural science laboratories there were cats with electrodes implanted in their brains and wires poking out of their skulls. By connecting an electric current and throwing a switch the cats would become snarling, spitting wild animals; by throwing another switch they became docile and fell asleep. I never got used to this spectacle and it put me off research using animals for good.

Chemical and food sensitivities give the impression of acting in a similar way. Families describe behaviour that is 'like throwing a switch'. Happy children can suddenly become screaming, sobbing and hysterical, frightening themselves as much as everyone else.

During exposure to chemicals, sensitive children can show dramatic changes in performance on standard psychological tests commonly used to screen children.

Auditory memory, in particular spontaneous recall, can be dramatically affected. It is not that the patient does not assimilate material he or she hears, but rather something interferes with his or her ability to use or recall that material when he or she wishes to do so.

Patients often say 'the information's in there but I can't get it out'.

Some patients suffer depression as their main symptom, others suffer changes in level of fatigue, anger and confusion.

The children with these problems can be rather hostile when they first come in for testing. Considerable work then has to be done to break down their defensive and often hopeless attitude. They lack self-esteem and feel they are useless and worthless. They are often particularly aware that they are the family's 'problem' and adopt the attitude that they might as well live up to their negative reputation.

Underneath this defensive facade is a very unhappy and confused child, desperate to be let out of an emotional and physical prison that his or her sensitivities have created.

Younger children are usually only too happy to take any drops prescribed which can help to mask reactions. At a follow-up appointment I asked one child I had tested if the drops had made him feel any different. His reply was intriguing: 'I like taking my drops, they take the bad out of me'.

Most children, even those on very strict diets which would discourage most adults, are remarkably compliant as breaches of the diet can have such upsetting consequeces physically and emotionally.

Sadly, as children get older the secondary emotional problems resulting from undiagnosed sensitivities become more deeply entrenched and their behaviour more maladaptive.

Realistically, if the first time parents bring their children for help is during adolescence then the prognosis is grim. Adolescents who have grown up with undiagnosed sensitivity are too angry and bitter with the world to easily accept help from professionals seen as authority figures in cahoots with Mum and Dad to control further their life and make it even more miserable.

They see parents, teachers, and life in general as letting them down. They feel they are not worth the effort. They have often never experienced contentment or pure joy, and literally don't know what they are missing.

Motivating such adolescents can be extremely difficult. Diagnosis and treatment must be directed through the children themselves. Parental support for dietary changes or direct help should only be given when requested by the child.

If you work through the parents of such children you risk alienating the child further and destroying whatever is left of the very fragile child/family relationship.

Other siblings and sometimes parents and teachers can have a vested interest in keeping a child a problem, and conscious and unconscious sabotage of his or her efforts to change have to be anticipated and recognised.

The child needs a great deal of support from outside the immediate family in order to change. It can be easier to stay with what you know rather than risk a new style that may have added responsibilities. Being 'born bad' or 'having a bad temper' lets you off the hook. But finding that Cola drinks, ice-cream, oranges and peanuts—your favourite foods—cause the problem puts you, the patient, in control.

'Getting better' syndrome demands adjustments by all the family. Suddenly the sick role is no longer appropriate and the modifications in behaviour and added responsibilities associated with being well can be quite frightening to someone who has become socially and emotionally 'out of practise' for many years. Younger children may never have had the chance to develop good work and study habits or social skills in the first place.

Most people are familiar with the end of holiday jitters as they gear up to return to work or school after a few weeks absence. Some people get these jitters even at the end of a weekend. So the nervousness and hesitancy of sensitivity patients, who may have been ill for months or years, at having to face everyday situations and responsibilities they have had to avoid for so long is understandable. Similarly, the child who became 'class clown' at school to avoid displaying his inability to cope with the work. The attention he has received in this role will be hard to do without, even if he can now do the work more easily. Teachers and parents need to give these children more constructive alternative roles which still provide recognition and attention. For instance, giving the 'class clown' a position of responsibility in the class and school over other children which is incompatible with behaving like a clown, but brings respect from the other children and attention from the staff.

One girl who was a constant source of frustration, friction and trouble on school buses, and who could very successfully promote 'subversive activities' against staff she did not like, was made a bus prefect even though she was only in Year 10. She was now in charge of many children, including some older than herself, but the new role of bus prefect was incompatible with getting the other children involved in bringing down authority figures. She became a highly successful prefect on a bus route renowned for its problems. The teachers she had effectively organised 'guerilla' tactics against were also able to breathe more freely as her more positive recognition extended into the classroom.

Another child who was extremely aggressive towards teachers and other students was able to discard his 'bully' role far more easily when his allergies were diagnosed by being put in charge of all new students to the school particularly the younger ones. It was his job to make sure *no one else* bullied them and to help them assimilate into the school's social structure.

# CHAPTER SIX

# Adults

Adults can find readjustment particularly difficult and families can become quite angry as roles in the family need to be reshuffled.

Often the allergic adult has become a very passive family member, too intent on struggling through each day's chores to be concerned with what children and spouse are up to. Once they start to feel better, patients often start to take a more active role in family affairs, giving their opinion freely and expecting it to be considered.

When one patient was diagnosed and started to feel better she said she felt like Rip Van Winkle waking up after a sleep lasting many years. She 'woke' to find the children nearly grown up and totally independent of her emotionally. The children and her husband had learnt a long time ago that they could expect little from her emotionally and only the bare essentials in a practical sense. She felt her presence was kindly tolerated but not really needed. In fact she soon realised that the friend who had been so supportive was her husband's mistress of many years standing, and he quite unashamedly admitted that he had coped with his wife's illness because of her support. The children were quite aware of Daddy's friend and had also come to rely on her a great deal.

The hardest thing was that the family firmly resisted her attempts to get actively back into their lives. She found herself desperately fighting for some sort of recognition in the family and sadly came to the conclusion that they had liked her best when she was sick and docile. Her eldest son didn't like being told that his smoking caused her mood changes, the daughter liked cooking and did not want Mum taking over her kitchen and her husband was certainly not going to give up his mistress. She found the family felt she had no right to comment on their clothes, behaviour, house decorating or where they would go for a holiday. Her suggestions were just ignored.

When she decided to leave she was devastated to realise that none of them were particularly upset or interested in maintaining contact.

Her illness, particularly because it had been misdiagnosed, had put her and her family through hell. The situation had placed intolerable strains on them as individuals and on their relationships.

Some of the most important and insidious secondary consequences of allergies/sensitivities in adults are due to misdiagnosis over many years.

Misdiagnosis leads to 'failed patient syndrome'. To understand much of the behaviour and emotional responses of these patients it is necessary to understand how this 'syndrome' develops, its symptoms and consequences.

## 'Failed patient syndrome'

'Failed patient syndrome' is an expression a patient and I devised to describe a problem that develops after misdiagnosis of any physical condition and in particular sensitivities.

The patient with a misdiagnosed organic disease (cancer, multiple sclerosis) will receive care and understanding when finally correctly diagnosed. However, even after an accurate diagnosis sensitivity patients still have a credibility problem with both health professionals and their families. They are still 'failed patients' as the diagnosis is unacceptable.

Much is written in textbooks for health professionals about the 'games' patients play and their attempts to manipulate the professional. However little is ever said about the 'games' that health professionals* also play.

Many health professionals unconsciously use a great deal of manipulation, aggression and arrogance to control their patients.

The aggression can be physical, as seen in the way they approach physical examinations of patients, or emotional, eg: asking intrusive questions which have no relevance to the problem at hand, making judgements, putting the patient in his or her place, etc. It may be verbal or non-verbal.

What patients don't realise is that when they consult a health professional they are actually playing a game—one with a tightly defined set of rules and an outcome in which there are supposed to be two winners. Health professionals want to succeed at curing you—this justifies their fees, makes them feel good, and confirms their belief in their own expertise. The patient wants to get better because that's the reason for the consultation, and because he or she has paid hard-earned money.

---

* *The term health professional is used throughout this discussion of 'failed patient syndrome' in its widest sense to include all health professionals treating patients (including medicos, naturopaths, dentists, psychologists, osteopaths, chiropractors, etc.)*

Everything proceeds very nicely in this game unless someone breaks the rules. Like all games, if somebody breaks a rule they are seen as cheats and others in the game become very angry and retaliate. Usually, for a patient with sensitivities, it is the patient who first breaks a rule. This is usually Rule No. 4—'The patient must get better'. Unlike other games, in this game the health professional is a participant and the referee as well. When this rule is broken the game can become particularly dirty, with intimidation, manipulation, aggression or arrogance being used by the health professional to regain control.

**Rules of the game**

1. The patient must have a clearly defined and easily diagnosed illness which can be cured by appropriately prescribed drugs, medication or treatment.
2. The patient must accept the diagnosis and treatment. 'The decision is final and no correspondence will be entered into.' The patient will carry out the treatment prescribed rigorously and to the letter. And if the patient dares to disagree with the diagnosis or treatment they will not argue about it.
3. The patient will adopt a suitably submissive role and will not argue, complain at being kept waiting, or object to interruptions by the phone or staff even though it is during the patient's consultation time. The patient must act as if they believe that they are not worth nearly as much as a human being as is the health professional.
4. *The patient will get better* and give all credit to the brilliant diagnosis and treatment. Furthermore, the patient will tell the health professional how grateful they are that the latter would condescend to make their relatively worthless body better.

Above all, the patient must not develop complications (unless they are of a nature which will without too much trouble further show the expertise and brilliance of the health professional). Also, the patient must never develop side effects to the treatment used as this undermines a basic rule—patients must get better not worse.

5. If after all efforts of the health professional to diagnose and treat the patient (usually about three to four visits) the patient isn't better then the patient must accept that their problem is either:
   (a) 'Stress'
   and/or (b) Neurosis
6. If 5. applies, the patient must not then ask what to do about (a) or (b) but must either:
   (c) See a psychiatrist
   (d) Live with their 'stress' or 'neurosis' and don't dare complain to the professional ever again.
   (e) Leave the practice and go bother someone else, preferably in another profession.

Really successful patients who are skilled players of the game get better within very few visits. These patients are usually seen as nice, pleasant people without any sign of neurosis.

People who are less skilled take longer to get better. These patients often evoke ambivalent feelings and are seen as suffering a certain amount of stress. Sometimes they are seen more positively as 'interesting cases'.

Bad patients are those that are no longer 'interesting cases', do not have clearly defined diagnoses, do not get better, have side effects to treatment, and have the audacity to keep coming back! They are seen as most definitely suffering 'stress' and are described as extremely neurotic. Smart bad patients stop going to the health professional. More obsessive types keep going and end up on anti-depressants, tranquilisers or both. All such patients end up with a diminishing bank balance and diaries full of appointments with various other health professionals.

Patients with food/chemical sensitivities are invariably 'failed patients' and develop the 'failed patient syndrome' which can have catastrophic consequences physically and emotionally.

Failed patients either just go home and put up with years of silent suffering, or start an appalling merry-go-round of health care professionals which inevitably gains them the label obsessive or hypochrondriac. Isolated from family and friends by their ill health, they get used to chronic discomfort and unaccountable mood changes. Slowly they adapt their lives to their condition. Some mothers adopt strategies to avoid lifting their babies and young children; they may breastfeed lying down as holding their baby may be too exhausting or too painful. Many give up breastfeeding altogether and resort to bottles propped up on a pillow. Just as allergic babies often can't bear to be touched, many allergic adults are the same. Cuddles from children become endurance tests, sex lives and affection are abandoned. They may only prepare meals they can cope with. It's frozen food because cutting, chopping and fiddly work like shelling peas causes pain in stiff fingers and joints.

Opening a gate on a cold morning requires a special effort for stiff fingers. Driving the car, leaning over and placing children in seatbelts may cause back pain. Pressing the seatbelt buckles is an effort causing more pain. The chronic discomfort leads to chronic irritability.

Appalling fatigue can mean 'clock watching' from mid-morning onwards desperately waiting for a tired spouse to relieve them. Instead of a cheerful homecoming, partners face a chaotic household and irritable whining children whose mother is, more often than not, close to tears or worse, sound asleep with the children left in cots—the only safe place she can leave them when fatigue and sleep overwhelm her.

Motherhood in the nuclear family is exhausting and demanding enough, but for the mother with sensitivities it can become a desperate hourly fight for physical and emotional survival.

The despair and guilt of mothers in this situation is horrific, made infinitely worse when they have no diagnosis other than 'bad mother', 'can't cope with life', 'spoilt and lazy' and 'post-natal depression'. I saw one lady who was diagnosed by a psychiatrist as suffering from post-natal depression for thirty-five years! Not only are they failed patients but usually they feel failures as mothers and wives as well. They feel incompetent in the most basic biological reason for their existence. Small wonder they often develop lasting emotional problems such as chronic depression and anxiety. Their relationships with their children often become distorted or break down altogether. Their marriages are brittle or break completely.

When one member of a family isn't coping or is ill it has a ripple effect on everyone else in the family and their relationships. Children feel cheated of effective parents, angry that their mothers let them down regarding something that they see as a basic right—the love, time, and attention of a mother who can meet their physical and emotional needs. The anger of these children is acute. Many switch off and dismiss their mothers as 'hopeless', others fight back trying to give as much hurt as they take.

As a therapist looking into these families there is often a chronic low grade depression in the whole family. Their emotional responses often appear dulled, there is no brightness or sharpness in their reaction to sadness or happiness. Life is joyless and montonous.

These families also repress feelings and emotions, frightened of what will be revealed if they dare let go. People walk on eggshells, frightened of upsetting the one who is ill.

When people say 'how are you?' people with sensitivities quickly learn that nobody really wants to know. Family and friends can be completely unaware of the degree to which the patient is suffering. If they do complain they tend to be labelled a neurotic, a whinger, moody or a hypochondriac.

Patients quickly learn the score. Complain and they are punished by family and friends with cold indifference or outright aggression: 'how dare you be sick and let us all down!'

Health professionals punish their failure to be good patients with a disbelieving, condescending attitude, scripts for tranquilisers or anti-depressants, or by total rejection: 'I think you should see a psychiatrist'.

Patients feel as if they are going through the motions of carrying out the chores of life without actually 'living'. They can somehow find the energy to do the bare essentials but there is nothing extra to give, no energy to experience life fully. Sensitivities can allow you to exist but rob you of the energy to live.

Waking, cooking, eating, cleaning become automatic responses but there is no joy, laughter, exhilaration, involvement or sharing.

The consequences for men (particularly if undiagnosed) can be equally catastrophic emotionally, physically and financially. Despite 'feminism', the fact remains that men are generally not allowed by their peers, and by our social expectations, to admit to physical symptoms or 'weakness'.

Thus the loneliness and isolation that sensitivity patients feel can be particularly acute for men. The secondary depression of the illness tends to be more serious as they are more threatened emotionally by being sick and are less likely to seek help.

Men especially, like to see themselves as strong, competent and in control at all times. Sensitivities can take their physical health and emotions beyond their control. They have difficulty discussing the lack of a definitive diagnosis which increases their anxiety and fear. Unlike women, who tend to withdraw and accept they are probably imagining the problems, men tend to either totally deny that they are sick and set about proving this to themselves, or they become extremely dependent. Of course these are generalisations and there are both men and women who accept and deal with their illness very well.

Either way, family relationships are severely strained. Wives, conditioned to expect their husbands to be physically strong and in control, often become extremely angry and frustrated with their husband's illness. They find it difficult not to show the frustration verbally and non-verbally as the illness can make a complete role reversal necessary—husband at home and wife the major breadwinner. To make this worse, the husband who has significant chemical sensitivities may be unable to do the shopping, use household cleaners, mow the lawn, etc. Many wives say they feel they would be better off as single parents—they feel their husbands are now just as demanding as their children.

Men, of course, sense the decrease in respect from wives, children, family and friends and become even more depressed.

It is vital that families discuss these issues openly and honestly. If they find they have negative feelings they cannot deal with then even one or two sessions with a psychologist as soon as possible after diagnosis can make an enormous difference to all the family in the long term.

Patients are initially extremely relieved to find there is a reason for their symptoms. However, this relief can be short lived as they tackle the practical problems of avoiding their allergens.

Life can become an endless battle to get special foods and water and to minimise chemical exposure. Sensitivities often cause acute social isolation, not just from friends but also from unsympathetic family members.

Because patients can look quite well, family and peers find it difficult to be sympathetic. Patients often feel they have to constantly justify their existence and illness and this can exacerbate symptoms as they attempt to 'prove' they are sick.

Parents suffer guilt feelings as they may be unable to fulfill expectations, eg: they can't attend school meetings because of the perfumes and aftershave lotions people use; or help with reading or other school activities because of the chemicals in the classroom. Their children become angry and frustrated and can learn very quickly how to take advantage of their parents' ill health.

The problems are made more difficult as sensitivity patients—like all chronically ill people—can develop significant psychological overlay to their symptoms, leaving patients further confused and their families and peers further frustrated and increasingly unsympathetic.

The consequences of a diagnosis of chemical sensitivity can be profound for the patient and his or her family.

The credibility of a diagnosis of chemical sensitivity can be seriously questioned if the diagnosis was made with unreliable testing methods or if psychological factors were not investigated or adequately considered.

Health professionals have a serious responsibility and ethical duty to their patients to make sure that any limitations of the testing are pointed out so that they can be taken into account when drawing conclusions.

If the diagnosis of sensitivities (particularly chemical) has been made by sublingual testing in conjunction with psychological assessment then it is possible to get a very clear picture of the degree of physical versus psychological factors operating.

Appropriate physical and psychological management of the problem can minimise many of the secondary psychological factors which can dramatically affect the patient's (and families') prognosis.

As the main treatment for sensitivities is avoidance, professionals diagnosing and treating these patients tend to place all responsibility for dealing with the illness on the patient or his or her family. With food sensitivity this may be a reasonable thing to do, but with chemical sensitivities it can be very unrealistic and place the family in terrible emotional conflict between the needs of a family as a whole and doing what a professional tells them they 'should do' for the sake of their child, spouse, etc.

The air we breathe can't be carved up into little packages and kept 'clean' by individuals. Food can be selected in supermarkets in its simplest and unprocessed form but the buyer has no real control over what chemicals have been used in the growing process. The fact is, *chemical sensitivity is a social problem.* Patients become the scapegoats when professionals make unrealistic demands on them as individuals or even use emotional blackmail to get them to follow instructions: 'You should do this for your child', 'Your child's future is at stake if you don't move to the country'.

Parents have come to me guilt-ridden and distraught because, for either financial or emotional reasons, they cannot carry out instructions given by health professionals regarding chemical avoidance. The guilt often changes to anger and frustration—not with the social system that allows such chemical contamination of the basic necessities of life—air, food and water—but with the patient him or herself. The family has been made a scapegoat by the professional and they in turn use the patient as a scapegoat. This conveniently avoids the real issue: why the hell are we allowing our food, water and air to become such health hazards?

It should be remembered that food/chemical sensitivity is fundamentally a very different process to most other illness in that enormous demands and responsibility are placed on the patient for both the diagnosis and management of the illness. The patient is actively involved. There are no magic blood tests, X-rays, etc. to test for sensitivities requiring only passive involvement by the patient. The patient cannot passively take a pill to make the illness better. At all times the patient must be actively involved and highly motivated (with the necessary financial resources for special food, water, filters, furnishings etc.). For this reason it can be impossible to diagnose and treat certain cultural groups or those with serious financial problems. If the patient sees the health professional's role as a healer and his or her own role as a grateful recipient, then satisfactory diagnosis and management is thwarted. Unfortunately, while the patient may be only too happy to take charge of his or her illness and be actively involved, the necessary assertiveness can be a real threat to a professional who then labels the patient 'difficult'.

As professionals treating these patients we can't have it both ways!

Patients need to look at the advice given not as a directive from 'God' (the doctor or other health professional) that must be carried out regardless, but in terms of their own emotional and financial situation.

Parents and spouses must recognise that sensitivities are a social problem and that there are real limitations on how much individuals can be expected to do. It is no good moving to the country (which may be more hazardous chemically than the city anyway) for the sake of one child if that means going on the dole and being isolated from the social and emotional support of family and friends. There are no guarantees that the child will be significantly better—particularly if the family is now emotionally stressed. For instance, one family moved to the country for the sake of one child with sensitivities and serious secondary emotional problems. Both parents gave up important careers which could not be pursued in the country and ended up on the dole. The two other children who were academically gifted gave up scholarships to private schools and music lessons. The child with sensitivities was only marginally better; one of the other children had enormous difficulty settling into the new environment, became extremely depressed and committed suicide.

This is an extreme example but it illustrates the need for families to *decide themselves what is best for the family as a whole*, regardless of what they are told may be technically physically ideal for a particular member.

The discussion so far has concentrated on individuals within families; however, a large number of adult patients are single with few emotional or financial resources. As with all illness, this group is at special risk of serious depression as they are often forced to battle on totally alone with an illness that may be invisible to others.

Satisfactory accommodation can become one of their biggest headaches as single people often need to share accommodation for financial reasons. It can be extremely difficult finding rental accommodation which is chemically 'safe', but getting the cooperation of others who are living in the same house regarding smoking, perfumes, hairsprays, air fresheners, etc. can be impossible.

Many single people who develop sensitivities are forced to return home to live with their parents, and this can place enormous strain on an otherwise good relationship. Parents may have great difficulty understanding the problem and treat the diet and chemical restrictions as 'a bit of a health fad', rather than taking the problem seriously.

Other parents are forced to become increasingly involved in an adult child's physical needs (special food, etc.). This can make parents feel very confused as their child is a mature adult and a dependent child at the same time.

The overriding emotions that all sensitivity patients and their families appear to feel are anger, frustration and guilt. Anger that their bodies seem to be letting them down and that meeting the most basic human needs—food, water, air and shelter—has suddenly become an extraordinary problem occupying ridiculous amounts of time and energy.

Frustration that no matter how careful they are, or how much responsibility they take for their illness, or what alternative treatment they seek, they still cannot control the quality of the air they breathe or the way their body reacts.

Guilt because professionals often make them feel they are not getting better because they are not doing everything they have been told to do strictly enough.

Understandably, if these feelings are allowed to run riot patients begin to see themselves as 'victims' with no control over their own lives. They can then develop an increasing chronic anxiety with periods of real panic.

In the workplace, food and chemical sensitivities are often mislabelled as 'stress symptoms' implying psychological stress. However, stress is experienced when a person's adaptive and coping abilities are exceeded by either physical or psychological demands (stressors).

Much has been written about the 'stress' of modern day living, and a lot of emphasis has been placed on emotional and psychological stressors. Frankly, I think it can be very much disputed that people are now experiencing more psychological stressors than at other times in modern history. But there is overwhelming evidence that since World War Two our bodies have been continually assaulted with a barrage of previously unknown physical stressors—chemicals in air, water and food (some five thousand new chemicals produced each year); electromagnetic radiation; changes in ultra-violet light conditions, etc., etc.—and no one has any real idea how these new physical stressors may be interacting with each other. For instance, it is now suspected that a change to polyunsaturated oil in the diet is increasing our vulnerability to ultra-violet light and the development of melanoma!

Before diagnosing a worker as suffering 'stress' (implying psychological stress), it's about time we started to ask what his or her physical stressors are as well. Especially as these physical stressors affect a person's ability to generally cope with life and work-related problems.

Patients are very familiar with being told they are 'suffering stress' by health professionals but feeling utterly bewildered as to what the psychological stress could be, especially if they like work and have a reasonable family life. A witch hunt can then start to try and discover a psychological stressor causing the problem and this can create more problems than are solved as the patient analyses his or her relationships to see what's wrong that he or she is unaware of.

Unfortunately, it just doesn't occur to most health professionals to ask about the physical environment in which the patients are working, and even when they do ask they are often ignorant as to the hazards in a fairly innocent looking office or workshop. In my opinion, people living in the western world in the 1980s have far more to fear from physical stressors than psychological stressors—particularly as they are unrecognised. One can't possibly cope with life's emotional stressors when the body is physically under siege and the mind is 'away with the fairies'.

# *PART THREE*

# *Prevention and Management*

# CHAPTER SEVEN

# *Minimising Chemical Exposure*

Prevention is always better than cure. In looking at the chemical environment that you as an individual can control the main ingredient is commonsense.

The degree of chemical exposure *you* can control around your home depends on:

(a) building design and structure
(b) chemicals brought into the home

## Building design and structure

Modern building design, structure and the materials used are now very different to those used in 'Grandma's Day' (see Table). Old housing design did of course have many drawbacks, particularly regarding use of natural light and heat, but modern house design needs to be reassessed in terms of the chemicals that the average home now contains.

| GRANDMA'S DAY | PRESENT HOUSING |
|---|---|
| No ducted central heating, heat only in living room/kitchen | Ducted heating circulating air from all areas of the house |
| High to very high ceilings | Low ceilings |
| Multiple wall vents | Fewer, if any, wall vents |
| Sliding or casement windows allowing good air flow | Top hung windows which restrict air flow |
| Subfloor space well ventilated as house built on stumps | No subfloor or poorly ventilated or completely enclosed subfloor |
| Wide and high central passage encouraging air flow throughout the house | Narrow low passages, winding through house often resulting in 'dead' air spaces |
| No pesticide spraying under, around or in house | Some councils demand spraying under house. Many householders have regular visits by pest controllers |
| Laundries and toilets in out-houses well separated from main house; most chemical cleaners were therefore away from living areas | Laundries and toilets inside house often adjacent to kitchen or en-suites off bedrooms. Chemical cleaners therefore inside house |
| Single garage totally separate from house and down back of yard | Multi-car garages and car ports attached to house |
| Wooden floors with rugs which could be removed outside to be shaken or washed | Fitted carpets with foam or rubber underlay—sometimes even in wet areas like bathrooms and kitchens and often on heated floors |

This brief comparison of older style and new housing gives an idea of the differences in house design which can contribute to poor ventilation and indoor air quality.

Of course, even in a well-designed house the quality of indoor air will also be determined by what is brought into the house and general housekeeping practices. Few people actually say they enjoy housework. Most of us would do anything to avoid it—so cleaners that promise to do the job for us more quickly and easily can be very attractive. Unwittingly, people can find their homes full of every conceivable cleaning product in an attempt to escape good old time-consuming 'elbow grease'.

## Chemicals brought into the home

The list of sources of natural and synthetic chemicals brought into and used around the home is daunting: cigarette smoke, heating, cooling and airconditioning systems, furnishings, building materials and finishes, clothing, water, floor coverings, toiletries, cleaners, pesticides, insecticides, herbicides, bedding, electrical and electronic appliances, packaging, etc.

Items that appear innocent, eg: plastic bags, can be continually 'gassing off' especially when heated. Even dry paint surfaces can give off fumes for many years after painting. In all discussions of chemical problems it must be stressed that the main problems in a particular home are highly individual and can be related as much to the site of the house, topography, local industries and the neighbours' incinerator, as to what is inside and outside the immediate home.

The guidelines given here are just that, and are based on my experiences with patients suffering predominantly psychological and behavioural symptoms. They are suggestions based on what is reasonable in a home without very costly and sometimes unnecessary alterations.

If you still suspect a problem after making these rudimentary changes and you have been diagnosed as chemically sensitive, don't get on a merry-go-round of further individual chemical tests but ask an indoor air chemist or architect to have a look at your house. It will be far more cost effective and helpful to you and your family's health in the long term. Long lists of 'failed' and 'passed' chemicals can be unreliable and can focus your attention too much on individual chemicals, ignoring unknown synergistic (combined) effects and much more significant problems in simple things like ventilation.

Very little is yet known about the effects of even common individual chemicals on human behaviour. The synergistic effects of these chemicals are a 'Pandora's Box'. From the little research that has been done it appears that these combined effects may be many times more potent than individual effects alone and, given the number of chemicals involved, impossible to research.

We can either decide that since the research is inadequate we will ignore the possibilities, or we can use some commonsense and start taking sensible precautions now.

There is a tendency to dismiss health hazards unless they cause cancer or immediate death and even then many people effectively tune out to the evidence. Allergies and sensitivities can cause death (note the dramatic increase in asthma in recent years) and a 'living death' for those seriously affected. Families can suffer an intolerable financial and emotional burden as well. For the majority, sensitivity can rob you of the ability to fully enjoy life and cause chronic subclinical ill health.

Before people embark on significant dietary restrictions they should take the following precautions to minimise chemical exposure.

## Water

### (i) Cooking and drinking

A good water filter is essential. Initially patients may buy a relatively cheap May Rei filter (about twenty-five dollars) which fits simply onto the kitchen tap for drinking and cooking purposes. However, if they can afford it, a filter such as a 'Mineral Pot' is a better long-term prospect and costs approximately a dollar a week to maintain. Many other filters are available which may be more suitable in individual situations. The Allergy Aid Centre has a very comprehensive range.

### (ii) Bathing

Until recently it was thought that water which was actually drunk was the potential hazard. However, there is now rather alarming evidence that bathing may pose a much bigger hazard, as many of the chemicals found in mains water can be more easily absorbed through the skin than first thought. The absorption is facilitated by soaps, detergents, etc.

Patients with serious sensitivities may well be advised to consider a filter on all mains water into their home.

Even people using rain water should use good quality filters as rain water is only as pure as the air the rain falls through, and the degree to which the roofing material itself is inert.

There is a tendency to blame the various Water Boards for these water problems but it may be that the difficulty of providing safe water in a bacterial sense make these chemicals necessary to some degree (flouride is another matter!). A water filter at the point of use (either the domestic supply or on each floor of a highrise building) may be the best compromise.

## Cigarette smoke

A smoker in the home can probably cause more problems than all the other sources put together and there is of course overwhelming evidence of the relationship between cigarette smoke and physical illness. Smokers have to face the fact that smoking in front of children is simply a sophisticated form of child abuse.

If a patient smokes it is often a waste of time and rather unfair putting pressure on other family members to cooperate with diets, special toiletries, etc., until the patient gives up smoking or at least cuts back.

If a patient has to live with a smoker relationships can become very strained. Fortunately, I find that once the problem is explained most smoking spouses or parents at least try to either give up completely, or restrict their smoking to outside or to one room of the house.

Some patients feel negative ion generators are helpful in getting small quantities of smoke pollution and other particles out of their air and settled onto surfaces. Ionisers really only help with comparatively large airborne particles. Patients have not found them helpful for chemicals (eg: perfumes, cleaners etc.).

If the patient lives with someone who says they just 'can't' restrict their smoking, then an air filter may be the only option. Although expensive they are much cheaper than a divorce or moving house! The Aironic 2000 costs about four hundred and fifty dollars and is excellent for moulds, cigarette smoke, dusts and general airborne pollution.

## Dust

Much publicity has been given to dust mite and asthma and this can be a very serious problem, however there are many other types of chemical dusts found in homes which for people with psychological symptoms can be a much bigger hazard. Ordinary vacuum systems tend to remove large dust particles (which tend to settle out of air anyway) but the very small dust particles usually pass through the filters in the machine and are released back into the room. It is these very small dust particles which are often the most hazardous.

Ducted vacuum cleaners are an excellent way of controlling dusts as the filters and dust collection system are outside the living area of the house. Steam cleaning carpets and furnishings with plain water by one of the very powerful cleaners where the motor is outside in a truck is an excellent way of ridding your home of a multitude of built up dust residues.

In terms of dust control, uncarpeted surfaces with natural fibre scatter rugs which can be washed are easiest. Don't 'dust' the house but damp wipe with plain water.

## Dust mite

Although there are various types of mites the individual with sensitivities needs to reduce overall exposure. They usually cause traditional allergy symptoms: wheezing, sneezing, and excema.

Dust mite tends to accumulate in bedding, bedroom carpets and soft furnishings. It is easier to control mites if a synthetic fill doona and pillow with *cotton* covers, pillows and sheets are used, rather than blankets and kapok filled pillows. Avoid fitted carpets and wipe floors and surfaces with cold tea solution (mites don't like the tannic acid). This can help with control, as does taking bedding outside and exposing to ultra violet light once a week. The room should be thoroughly vacuumed, including mattresses, at least once a week.

## Obvious chemicals

For example, cleaners, toiletries, cosmetics, etc.

### (i) Inside the home

If looking for obvious chemicals in your home, the first place to start are kitchen, bathroom and laundry cupboards.

The best way to start this sort of clean-up is to remove every cleaner, toiletry, hairspray and mousse, cosmetic, pest strip, deodoriser, pressure can, soap powder, stain remover, boot polish, polishing cloths and polishes, mothballs, etc. to the garage and start again!

The overall chemical exposure can be drastically reduced in the home by using alternative products. Included here are some better alternatives but people need to read labels carefully and check that a product is acceptable for them individually.

For general cleaning and toiletries 'Herbon' have developed a range of petrochemical free products in conjunction with the Australian Allergy Association and specialists in the field of environmental medicine. The range includes laundry, kitchen, bathroom and toiletry products and is generally available at health food stores. Herbon's products are about as 'allergy free' and environmentally safe as is practically possible. They have also recently researched and developed new herbal extracts which now make possible petrochemical-free hair conditioner, anti-dandruff shampoo and non-aluminium roll-on deodorant.

Some of the laundry products use eucalyptus oil so people who have turpene sensitivity should be careful.

Amway and Swipe are good brands with a range of toiletries and cleaners.

Old fashioned 'White Lily' and bicarb. of soda are excellent for sinks, troughs and bathrooms.

Fridges and Freezers—Bicarb. of soda solution (2 tspns to 600 ml of water) absorbs odours and is good to wipe out fridges and freezers.

Furniture Polish—Use olive oil or other vegetable oil

All Purpose Cleaner—'Biotique' is a totally petrochemical-free herbal product which is quite outstanding, particularly with metal surfaces (silver, brass, etc.).

Toiletries—Herbon, Amway, Swipe, Mill Creek shampoo, Blackmores, Aloe Vera, plain soaps such as Velvet, Simple Soap, Castile

—Toothpastes such as Red Seal, Herbal and Blackmores or plain bicarb. of soda and salt mixture

—Suntan lotions can be difficult as they use PABA

derived from a petrochemical, as the sunscreen. However, Herbon have now developed a 15+ totally petrochemical-free sunscreen using a new herbal extract

Cosmetics—Blackmores, Nutrimetics, Clinique, Nature's Way

Moulds—Wipe the surfaces (eg: showers, window sills, skirting boards, blinds etc.) with vinegar

Pantry—Wipe surfaces with bicarb. soda solution or, if moulds are a problem, with vinegar

Windows—Swill half a teaspoon of Swipe Concentrate around and out of a spray top container. Refill container with water. Alternatively, a teaspoon of vinegar in 1.5 litres of hot water

Clothes—Living on a muddy farm I find heavily soiled and children's clothes are best left to soak several hours in laundry powder (Herbon, Amway, Swipe). I use an old washboard, a hard brush dipped in plain Velvet soap, bicarb. of soda or borax and plenty of elbow grease to scrub the clothes before transferring to a washing machine for rinsing. This may sound primitive but I've decided it's better than having my son covered in excema.

—For normal machine washing use one of the previously suggested laundry powders. Bicarb. soda or borax can be rubbed on particularly dirty spots.

Insecticides and Pesticides—Firstly buy a fly swat! Make sure fly screens fit properly. Secure all openings into the house from rats, mice and possums. A vacuum cleaner is an excellent pest trap if there are large numbers of flies or a runaway mouse.

—Eucalyptus oil wiped on surfaces is good for controlling moths, silverfish and ants. Similarly, lavender oil or lavender sachets among clothes.

Note: Turpene sensitive people will need to be very careful with eucalyptus and lavender.

For specific problems contact:

Total Environment Centre
18 Argyle Street
Sydney NSW 2000
Ph: (02) 27 8476 or 27 4714

Please note that there may be other petrochemical-free and low allergy products available of which I am unaware. The above recommendations are based on my own and my patients' experience.

**(ii) Outside the home**

Here the biggest hazards are the garden itself and the garage/workshop containing the car and the chemicals you just got rid of from inside the house!

Go around the garage and ask yourself: Do I really need this particular chemical, spray, pesticide, etc.? If the garage is attached to the house and near windows that would take chemical fumes into the house be particularly ruthless or perhaps use a little gardening shed well away from the house (but not near your neighbour's house!).

Household incinerators are now recognised as one of the biggest contributors to air pollution and the sooner they are banned the better. There are much better ways of disposing of rubbish—composting, bottle collections and the municiple tip. Get rid of your incinerator.

Throughout this book the emphasis has been on sensitivities. However, the extremely toxic chemicals used by pest controllers and the routine spraying often demanded by councils raise the question of the outright toxic effects which may arise from these chemicals. If your home has been sprayed outside or inside then find out what chemicals were used. If you are concerned by what your enquiries reveal, consult the experts for an assessment of your home (eg: the Toxic and Hazardous Chemicals Committee).

## Packaging

Next time you buy your groceries consider the type of material in which they are packaged. If possible, buy goods packaged in glass or cellophane. This is especially important for meat and dairy produce. (Some types of plastic packaging are not a problem in terms of food contamination but unless you are a plastics chemist it's impossible to tell which are acceptable.)

Store foods in glass. It really is possible to live without plastic cling-wraps! Wrap school lunches in cellophane bags. Don't store plastic bags in the house, especially near heat sources such as dishwashers or under the sink where the 'gassing off' will be exacerbated.

## Clothing and bedding

When you consider that our bodies are in constant close contact with clothing and bedding it makes good sense to consider the chemicals that may be given off from these as they are heated by your body.

Patients mention feeling giddy and 'fuzzy' while ironing clothes, particularly synthetics. Cotton bedding and cotton, silk or wool clothing are the most chemically free, although some people find wool irritating. There is now a fashion swing back to natural fibres so even cheap clothes and bedding can be found without too much difficulty for adults. With children the problem is more difficult as synthetic mixtures can be more hardwearing so they tend to be used in children's clothes. Unfortunately, school uniforms are nearly always synthetic.

Waterbeds can be a particular hazard for the sensitive person as the heater causes a steady vapourisation of the liner which then envelops the sleeper. Rubber hot water bottles can also produce a rather potent brew. Electric blankets are not advisable owing to the possible harmful effects of electromagnetic radiation.

Some patients need to go to the extreme of special mattresses—avilable at the Allergy Aid Centre. Generally, a good thick cotton or wool mattress overlay on normal synthetic mattresses is sufficient, but not if they have been treated for moths.

As few of us can afford to throw out clothes and bedding it may take some time to change these items to better alternatives but the sooner the better, especially with children.

## Heating, cooling and cooking

This is an area in which it is almost impossible to generalise as each fuel source has its own special potential problems. All fuel sources for heating and cooking need to be working as efficiently as possible with the absolute minimum of combustion biproducts. In the home, electric fuel sources tend to be the cleanest.

Ducted systems can be a problem as they may circulate hazards throughout the house rather than allowing them to remain isolated in one room, eg: cigarette smoke.

Airconditioners must be well maintained and appropriate in size and type for what they are expected to do.

## Light

This of course is not a 'chemical' hazard in the home but there is increasingly well documented research (particularly from Eastern Europe) to show that light quality can have a dramatic effect on mood and physical health. I find this appears to be particularly so in women and a number of patients have commented on the difference that even skylights have made to their mood and general feeling of well being. Before putting in skylights though, tackle the chemicals and your diet!

## Moulds

Even new houses can have serious mould problems. Moulds tend to grow most in damp, poorly lit and poorly ventilated areas like bathrooms, kitchens, laundries, under floor coverings, in cupboards and behind curtains. If your house has mould problems look at drainage outside the home to make sure water runs away from the house—especially where the house is on a slab cut into a clay soil. Check that earth is not up against walls above the floor level and that damp courses are working properly.

Mould growth can be controlled by improving ventilation in the area affected (eg: exhaust fans, preferably vented outside) and increasing light. Painting rooms in light rather than dark colours can dramatically affect light conditions without making structural changes. Keep climbing plants, shrubs and trees clear of windows. Collect falling leaves and clear away rotting vegetation—but compost don't burn! Make sure any leakages or breaks in pipes are properly repaired and the area thoroughly dried out.

## Ventilation

Inadequate ventilation can be a serious problem. Modern homes tend to have few wall vents to the outside. Flues and wall vents should be vented to the outside not to wall cavities or ceiling space. The trend towards top hung windows severely restricts air movement in and out of the house, unlike the older casement or sliding windows.

Narrower passageways and smaller rooms with low ceilings further restrict air movement.

With airconditioning and ducted heating many homes have windows and doors tightly closed to outside air, particularly if both adults in the house work away from home.

Patients who complain their symptoms are worse in winter are often those with a house that is effectively sealed off from fresh air for many months of the year.

Check there is good ventilation in, around and under the house. Try and open the whole house to fresh air (propping doors and windows wide open and using fans if necessary) for at least an hour each day.

The Egyptians entombed the dead—don't entomb the living!

## Hobbies and businesses at home

To try and reduce overheads there are increasing numbers of people working from home and undertaking hobbies using toxic materials.

Careful attention should be given to where any work or hobbies using such materials are located (eg: paints, fibreglass, glues, solders, etc.). If possible, work in an area well separated from the main house and with its own ventilation and heating system.

Old newspapers and magazines, art materials, plastic bags, etc. should be kept outside the house when not being used. One patient actually slept in the same room as her wet oil canvasses.

## Owner builder/renovators

The dramatic rises in home prices over the last ten years and relaxing of regulations have created a large number of hard working and enthusiastic owner builder/renovators.

These owners and their young children often live in appalling conditions for months, sometimes years, while they build or renovate their house.

The high costs involved means that the building programme is often stop/start depending on weather, funds and other work and family commitments. This can result in the whole family being exposed to very hazardous building and painting materials in a way that was never intended by the manufacturers of such materials.

Owner builders are usually under considerable stress, often eating hasty and erratic meals prepared under very difficult circumstances. This combination of prolonged emotional and physical stress, poor nutrition and prolonged exposure to toxic materials can be disastrous for the health of the whole family (including their pets). Pregnant women need to be especially careful. Pregnancy is not the time to become a house painter!

If you are an owner-builder then be extremely careful with the materials you use, how they are stored, and how you dispose of left-over materials.

Try to build or renovate to completion one room or section of the house at a time. Even if this means living in one room it will make it easier to keep raw building materials and glues, paints, insulation, etc. away from where you are actually living.

Seal the completed section off from the section still being built. Wide packaging tape can seal doors and windows very effectively. If necessary, use a fan to control air flow so that the living section draws fresh air and not air from the part-built area.

In damp or humid conditions it is more effective to close all windows and doors and 'cook' fresh paint with a heater left in the room for a couple of days. When the paint is quite dry then open all the windows and doors to get rid of the fumes. Stay out of the room until the paint is completely dry.

Choose all materials carefully and follow manufacturer's directions exactly. There are now a large range of industrial masks available for reducing exposure to dusts and chemicals.

Avoid routine spraying for ants, etc. under slabs and raised floors. If necessary, challenge the local council's regulations on spraying. Information on alternative methods of pest control is available from the Toxic and Hazardous Materials Committee.

Do not burn off-cuts of timber, particle board, plastic pipe, insulation and wiring. Most timber for housing, particularly pine, is treated with a variety of chemicals. *Never ever* burn such materials in fireplaces or stoves inside the house.

Do not make the mistake of thinking that natural materials are necessarily safest. Timber is often treated with chemicals at the mill as well as being stained and sealed in the home. Many chemical treatments on timber cannot be detected by sight or smell. Straw ceiling batts are treated with mould inhibitors.

Wool carpets can be a problem if 'mothproofed' and sprayed with soiling inhibitors.

In very general terms, plaster walls painted with good quality paints, brick and stone walls and hard flooring tend to cause minimal problems once the building is finished.

Keep children and pregnant women well away from the area being built and away from paints and materials being stored.

(*A-Z Chemicals in the Home* is a comprehensive book which gives an excellent overview of the alarming nature and extent of chemicals to be found in the average home.)

## Babies

Most parents like to spend time decorating the baby's room but if painting is to be done, do it as far ahead of the birth as possible with good quality paint.

Don't prolong painting time unnecessarily by doing it in stages. Get the job over and done with as soon as possible.

If you are an allergic/sensitive mother or have a strong family history of allergy make sure that you visit the hospital and let them know of any special requirements you may have well in advance, particularly regarding medications and analgesics. Take a portable water filter into the hospital.

Maternity hospitals are becoming increasingly mother and baby orientated in their thinking which makes them much more receptive to your views than before. But do remember that the indoor air quality issue is a new one so that staff may not be aware of much of what you are talking about. Give them this book to read if necessary.

Maternity ward and administrative staff have been particularly concerned and helpful to my patients with significant sensitivities, and even if they have not fully understood they have made every attempt to respect the mother's wishes.

Of course as there are three shifts per day in hospitals it can be difficult for every single staff member to know your requirements so labelling the baby's cot with 'allergic mother' or 'family history of serious allergy' can alert them to the possibility of problems.

If you do have to bottle feed try to use glass bottles that are boiled and not chemically sterilised. The water to make up the formulas needs to be filtered and boiled.

Be very careful with the furnishings for a baby's or a child's room. Keep the room simple, using natural fibres and hard floorings with scatter rugs which can be washed. Soft toys are usually foam or synthetic filled. They can be difficult to wash making them perfect harbourers of dust mite. Many soft plastic toys for babies are extremely 'smelly' and offensive even to adults.

## Pets

Special care should be taken when pets live or spend large amounts of time inside the home. Dog and cat allergies are extremely common. Some people are bothered greatly by birds, particularly pigeons. By making sure that dogs and cats have their own basket and bedding and are not allowed to roam on the furniture and in bedrooms dander and mite problems can be minimised. Try and restrict animals to one room with hard flooring and ensure that they are properly house trained.

Don't allow children to cuddle or pet animals that are wearing flea collars or have just been bathed in chemicals to kill fleas.

Pets are wonderful for children and adults but strict hygiene needs to be observed for the sake of the animal as well as its owner.

# Away from home

Patients and their families may have some control over their own home and garden plot but at kinder, school and work the problems can be much more difficult to tackle.

The work environment is extremely complex depending on what sort of work is being carried out and under what conditions. If you have significant sensitivities then the workplace needs to be considered on an individual basis to see what is realistically possible. Occupational health and safety officers from the unions have access to a wide range of resources and should work in with health practitioners.

Before approaching your child's kinder or school make sure you have already made realistic modifications at home. For instance, asking teachers not to wear perfume when you are a chain smoker is not going to endear them to your cause!

Rather than waiting for your child or somebody else's to get sick, bring up the issue of chemicals in the indoor and outdoor environment at parent committee meetings and school council meetings.

Approach the teachers first. They are in the front line dealing with behaviour and psychological symptoms *en masse* in their classes. I have found they are usually only too pleased to look at anything which might explain and help some of the extremely difficult behaviour and learning problems they have to do battle with on a daily basis.

Alert teachers to the hazards already discussed regarding home environments which are also applicable to schools. Kinders and schools also have to consider their storage and use of materials and chemicals in the classroom and around the schoolgrounds (spirit pens, cleaning materials, freshly printed material, art material, glues, gas heaters, gas and chemicals in science rooms, plastic and synthetic furnishings, toiletries and clothing worn by thirty or more warm bodies in one room, herbicides sprayed on playing fields and paths, vapourising asphalt, etc.).

Teachers and parents can actually do a great deal towards reducing the overall level of chemical exposure. Before deciding on new uniforms, buying new equipment or furnishings stop and think whether you have chosen the best possible alternative from a chemical point of view.

For some years I have recommended parents with sensitive children send their children to a particular kindergarten which was fairly sound from a chemical point of view and had staff who were very willing to fit in with what a 'sensitive' child needed. I was appalled to find one year that the parents committee had decided against the recommendations of the kinder teacher and had replaced the hard vinyl floor (which was practical and very satisfactory chemically) with a 'nice new synthetic carpet' throughout the building. They also replaced the safety glass beakers with soft plastic beakers!

In finding likely sources of chemical exposures in and around buildings a very useful guide is the 'sniff test', ie: use your nose! If you can smell an object then it is gassing off some kind of chemical so seek out the least 'smelly' alternative. Some very nasty chemicals are actually invisible and odourless but the sniff test is a good guide to more obvious hazards.

For instance very hard plastics are extremely 'inert' which means they have virtually no odour. This makes them very satisfactory for children's toys. Soft plastics often have a distinct odour indicating they are 'gassing off'.

Similarly 'hard' vinyl tiles have very little odour compared to the soft cushioned vinyls.

Parents and teachers report that many children can be fussy about whose car they will travel in, whose house they are happy to go to and which people they will allow physically close. This of course can be the usual separation anxiety that normal children have to some degree, but 'sensitive' children have often told me they find the 'smell' of certain teachers, children, homes and cars highly offensive and upsetting.

It is worth remembering that children these days are exposed to the effects of chemicals long before they are born. Every attempt should be made to keep chemical exposure to a realistic minimum.

Besides these major considerations there are many other 'details' (eg: furnishing materials, packaging, topography etc.) which contribute to air quality and chemical sources around the home. In this chapter I have discussed the major problems which I have found can be realistically tackled by individuals and families. Except in extreme cases, these measures are sufficient and cost effective. If further measures need to be taken they must be done on an individual basis, with a site inspection to avoid very costly errors.

CHAPTER EIGHT

# Dietary guidelines

## During pregnancy

The importance of diet in minimising the chances of developing sensitivities starts before a woman becomes pregnant.

Women who have undiagnosed sensitivities causing significant physical symptoms need to have their own sensitivities properly diagnosed and managed before they become pregnant. Pregnancy causes changes in the functioning of a woman's immune system so she will not reject her baby as a 'foreign body'. During or just after pregnancy, women can find sensitivity symptoms changing. Especially after delivery symptoms can become much worse or be actually 'triggered' for the first time.

Pregnancy and looking after a baby can be physically and emotionally demanding enough without the added burden of a sick mother or child.

For women without known sensitivities (and particularly those with a history of allergy) it is a good idea to take special care to eat as wide a variety of foods as possible and aim to have no particular food more than two to three days per week (see 'Dietary Guidelines' in this chapter).

A varied diet stops the baby becoming overexposed to

particular foods before birth. Overexposure before birth can create major sensitivities in susceptible infants. Mothers who are vegetarians need to be especially careful as their diet is often high in milk products and wheat—two of the most common allergens.

Water is one of the most common sensitivity problems and as mentioned earlier it is a good idea to use a good water filter for all cooking and drinking water.

Food needs to be as fresh and unprocessed as possible. If you live near a genuine organic or biodynamic food store then you can further reduce your intake of chemicals. However, don't start driving long distances in heavy traffic to get organic or biodynamic food as any chemical advantage will be lost by the chemical exposure in the car and traffic!

Be particularly careful if you find yourself developing aversions or addictions to certain foods during pregnancy as it is likely that these are the foods to which you are sensitive. Try eliminating a 'binge' food out of your diet for a week. You may well find after a difficult few days of 'withdrawal' that your general health improves and you lose the desire to binge.

The desire to binge can also be minimised by going for a long hard walk instead. This can trigger the body's own endogenous opiate system and reduce the cravings for a food. Do not do hard aerobic exercises unless you are used to it and even then only in moderation. Pregnant women should avoid doing any exercise or activity which raises body temperature.

## Infants

Once you have your baby make every attempt to breastfeed. The best way of minimising sensitivities in a child is to breastfeed exclusively for at least the first six months and to continue breastfeeding for at least twelve months. The pros and cons are excellently covered in Maureen

Minchin's book, *Breast-Feeding Matters*, which is well worth reading if you have any doubts.

Some babies, despite the variety of foods in the mother's diet and exclusive breastfeeding still develop sensitivities causing distressing symptoms (eg: colic, diarrhoea, constipation, rashes, general irritability or repeated infections. In some babies the only apparent sign of sensitivity may be a red ring-like rash around the anus (anal ring). In other babies, a clue may be 'milk rash' which looks like adult acne and if severe may cover most of the body.

Before stopping breastfeeding it is worth keeping strictly to the dietary guidelines which follow and recording a symptom diary to see if an association can be made with a food in the mother's diet. This is often quite a successful method with young babies. Reactions to breast milk tend to occur within minutes if related to a medication the mother is taking, or within two to four hours if a food. It is easier if you simplify your meals during this time without sacrificing your nutritional needs—eg: instead of muesli, which is a mixture of grains, have just Weeties or Rice Bubbles or oats; instead of three to four different vegetables every day, have just one or two (but more of each vegetable).

It should be remembered that sensitivities are very individual and generalisations such as 'cabbage gives a baby wind' may not be a very reliable or useful guide. The foods most likely to cause problems, particularly where there is a family history of allergy, are—milk, wheat, eggs, oranges, tomatoes, peanuts, yeasts, and tap water and of course any product containing these foods.

Don't bother trying to eliminate foods unless your diet is basically sound, with no additives or stimulants, and you are not smoking. If you decide you need to eliminate these foods from your diet then seek the help of a clinical nutritionist or dietician.

If the baby is still having problems or the mother is on medication then there may be no choice but to try a formula. Most formulas available in hospital are milk-based. Enfalac is a formula designed for premature or low birthweight babies and is particularly high in milk proteins. As milk proteins are thought to be the main cause of milk allergy reactions it may be necessary to discuss this choice with your paediatrician if there is a strong history of milk allergy in the family.

For normal full-term babies, the choice is between milk-based formulas (S26, SMA, Simulac, Nan, Lactogen, Enfamil, Delact Infant, Digestelact) and soy-based formulas (Prosorbee, Isomil and Infasoy). In S26 and Nan the milk protein is artificially 'modified' and this can make them less of a potential problem regarding allergies. Prosorbee contains no sucrose and since sucrose is also a common cause of sensitivities is probably the better choice of the soy formulas. Babies brought up on soy formulas, especially from an early age, can develop sensitivities to soy so care needs to be taken when introducing other legume foods (beans, peas). Delact for infants under six months and Digestelact for infants over six months are milk-based but have been modified so that they are very low in lactose.

Babies or children with severe sensitivities sometimes need to be put on special formulas containing predigested protein which makes them less likely to cause problems and more easily absorbed by a sensitive digestive system. The most well known brands are Nutramigen, Pregestimil and Alfare.

Changing formulas can be difficult while the child gets used to a different taste. It often helps to stop all solid foods until the new formula has been accepted. Making the formula into ice-blocks can make it a more interesting food to a child and the coldness tends to diminish the strange taste. This works just as well with older children switching from cow's milk to soy milk. The milk is even more palatable first time by making fruit 'smoothies', eg: banana, apricot, pineapple. Serve very cold with fruit juice ice-blocks.

Solids are better not introduced until six months of age. Foods are best introduced one at a time and a record of foods introduced and any symptoms kept so that any reactions are properly recorded. It is very easy to forget if the symptoms are mild. Some professionals suggest having the same food for three or four days to see if it is 'safe'. However in susceptible children this may actually 'sensitise' them. I usually suggest parents introduce a new food for a day and then wait to see if any reactions occur over the next three days. If 'safe', then reintroduce the food on the fourth day. This is called a four-day rotation. Although it may seem slow and tedious, care and time taken with introducing solids can reduce sensitivities to a minimum. Continue testing foods and arrange the diet on this four-day rotated basis, ie: a particular food is only eaten once every four days.

It is best to start introducing solids with vegetables (zucchini, squash, pumpkin, carrots, peas, cauliflower, sweet potato, broccoli, potato etc.). Next introduce fruits (pears, apples, banana, apricots, peaches etc.), then meats such as lamb, free range chicken, beef and finally grains. Start with the gluten free grains (rice, tapioca, millet) then barley, rye and wheat.

If foods have been introduced slowly there may be no reason to introduce grains until twelve months of age or more when the immune system of the digestive system is more mature and less likely to become sensitised.

Where there is a history of family allergy, cow's milk, wheat, oranges, nuts, egg white, tomato and yeast (eg: Vegemite) are best left until after twelve months of age.

If syptoms do develop to a food then eliminate the food and try it again in a few weeks. Remember, a baby's digestive system has to develop and may tolerate certain foods later.

If the child has symptoms which appear to change as they get older, eg: eczema changing to repeated ear infections changing to asthma then there is probably a hidden food allergy/sensitivity contributing.

It is important that the foods introduced are as fresh and unprocessed as possible otherwise a food may be classed as a problem when a food additive is the real culprit.

## Children and adults

Children's parties and social gatherings can be a nightmare for food sensitive children and adults. Many patients find that if they are extremely strict at home they can cope with the odd party without too much trouble. Some find that taking Vitamin C and B Complex or Buffered C (before they indulge) minimises symptoms. After all, life is for living! (Buffered C is a mixture of Calcium, Magnesium and Potassium carbonates with Vitamin C) and is available in health food shops under the Microgenics label or on mail order from Nutricology, PO Box 191, Corio, 3214.

Some patients however have severe reactions and in these cases they may be forced to take along their own food or water or let the hostess know well in advance of their limitations.

Unfortunately for sensitivity patients, offering and sharing food and drinks are fundamental social graces woven into the simplest occasions. People naturally feel rejected if they offer food and/or drink (even tea or coffee!) and a guest refuses—especially if the hosts have not been warned and have gone to a lot of trouble to prepare or buy food.

If sensitivity patients must adhere to a strict diet when socialising they need to be very assertive with friends and hosts in advance wherever possible. Friends and family are often only too relieved and pleased to be given definite alternatives that they can provide, eg: herb tea, safe fruits attractively presented. Even formal dinner parties can be acceptable to host and patient with a little forethought. The hostess may be able to use your permissable foods as a 'skeleton' for the actual meal, eg: avocado, lamb, beans, sweet potato, bananas, almonds, may all be 'safe' foods which the hostess can expand on for other guests without making your meal too obviously different.

It is up to sensitivity patients to use some social sensitivity in the way they talk about their health problems and with whom. Patients who have accepted their illness and restrictions and quietly 'get on with it' are accepted very well by friends, family and peers.

The fact is that food/chemical sensitivity is extremely threatening to other people. All illness tends to be threatening to others but food/chemical sensitivity forces people to face head on the prospect that we are losing control over our environment—and control of our environment is a goal ruthlessly pursued by most modern societies.

Patients must use commonsense and consideration when wanting to discuss or complain about their illness. The time, situation, and the listener need to be appropriate. In social gatherings as people realise your diet is 'different' there is a natural curiosity and they may actually ask questions and be genuinely concerned. However for your own sake it is often far more prudent and tactful to joke about it or change the subject otherwise the hostess can find herself watching her guests suspiciously looking at the food she has prepared and the furnishings of her home as suddenly potential enemies. The evening can suddenly become very flat!

There is a time to campaign your cause, complain bitterly and express your fury without boring everyone you know and turning them away from you and your cause.

Adults usually have enormous difficulty accepting long-term dietary and social restrictions even if their health does improve. A patient who is also the household cook can find preparing food that he or she can't eat a subtle form of torture—they buy it, cook it, touch it, see it, feel it, smell it, even hear it, but they can't eat it!

It is little wonder then that children can find the restirctions intolerable—although it is amazing how compliant and sensible young children can be compared to adults!

If your child has restrictions it is vital that they see the restrictions not as some awful health fad of Mum's, or some new subtle form of punishment designed for them and no one else in the family.

Before even considering eliminating any 'normal' food (eg: milk, wheat etc.) look at the chemical load in your home (see previous chapter) talk to your partner, and discuss following the general dietary guidelines. If your partner can't do without their Mars Bars or junk food make an agreement that they indulge away from home. If your partner is totally unconvinced that it is worthwhile ask if they will at least support you with the diet in front of the children for a set period of time—say four weeks on general dietary guidelines and a further four weeks if other restrictions become necessary. Gaining cooperation for a set finite time can be much easier. If there has been considerable improvement by the end of that time, your partner is usually happy to continue.

When changing the family's diet it is a good idea for both parents to sit down with the children and explain why the changes are being made. This forces you to get a very clear idea in your own mind of what you are doing and why. Instead of letting the family think it's your latest funny idea, refer to the 'experts': psychologist, doctor or other health professional. Tell the family you have paid a lot of money to consult the expert and it is your responsibility as a parent to feed them as well as possible. Explain that you feel you would be negligent if you allowed them to eat things the 'experts' said were doing them harm. Children react well to the authority of experts (until they are teenagers anyway) and can certainly (often begrudgingly) see that as a parent you have a responsibility to do what is best for them physically. Don't ask permission of your child to make the changes—as a parent and breadwinner and cook it is your right to decide what they eat. Tell them what the changes will be and say you are going to review the diet in, say, four weeks. If birthdays or special occasions are coming up then explain these occasions are special and they can eat what they like for that meal.

Once you have discussed the dietary guidelines place the diet (preferably typed on 'official' looking stationary) on the fridge door.

I always discuss a diet with the child even if very young and make it very clear that I am telling their mother what she has to feed them. I give them the diet sheet on my letterhead so that it is quite clear whose 'funny idea' the diet has been.

This helps when the child is demanding a food they had previously been allowed. Simply point to the diet sheet and say 'the list says we can't have that food'. In this way Mum appears controlled by the list too. One six-year-old patient stopped his tantrum after being told this. He quietly looked at the list for some time. He then turned to his mother working at the kitchen sink and exploded: 'Then change the bloody list'!

To make it easier on all the family's will power remove all items from the pantry and freezer not allowed on the diet (read labels!)—processed cheeses, biscuits, sugar, white flour, packet mixes, canned foods (except those allowed), cakes, lollies, soft drinks, pizza, croissants, etc. Give them away or ask a friend to store them. Go for a tour of the best greengrocer you can find and really look at the incredible variety of fruits and vegetables that are now available. Most people shop in a hurry and automatically go for the potatoes, peas, beans, carrots, lettuce, tomato and apples without ever really seeing all the other fresh foods available.

It is no good embarking on such a diet, though, if your

home is a chemical hazard. Chemical sensitivity particularly affects behaviour and a chemical cleanup needs to be done before starting the diet.

Don't panic, I don't mean pulling the house to bits but look at the ways of minimising chemical exposure carefully: I have often had patients who had family members working in the cleaning industry whose houses were literally chemical soups of every conceivable cleaner imaginable—often of industrial strength.

Sick patients have often found significant relief, particularly with fatigue symptoms, by simply getting rid of these cleaners.

## Dietary guidelines

These guidelines are for people wishing to improve their general health or those suspicious that foods may be contributing to their symptoms. The first two to three weeks can be difficult as you adjust to a different diet and 'withdraw' from foods to which your biochemistry has adapted.

It may seem hard work but cut out forbidden foods completely rather than reduce your intake slowly. Although the first couple of weeks can be very difficult your body quickly adjusts and you can actually develop a healthy aversion to the forbidden foods particularly salt and sugar.

Most patients feel so much better after following this diet strictly for four weeks that they have no trouble sticking to it as a daily routine. On special occasions or when out they may relax the restrictions but many find the unpleasant consequences not worth it.

Smokers who have tried unsuccessfully to give up have found that giving up is easier once their diet has been modified and they have reduced their exposure from other chemicals in the home. Smokers can get relief from nicotine withdrawal symptoms by taking the Buffered C mentioned earlier.

The main aim of the diet is to remove additives, processed foods and stimulants from the diet and replace them with fresh simple unprocessed foods, and to increase the range of foods eaten. Check at your children's school to make sure the school canteen is not undermining all your efforts. If necessary, campaign to change the foods sold. Frankly I think it's time that 'Teacher Support Services', which helps schools with programmes for children with learning and/or behavioural problems, considered blackbanning those schools who refuse to remove junk food from the canteen.

Withdrawal symptoms (nausea, diarrhoea, constipation, arthralgia, myalgia, headaches, irritability) may make you feel initially worse rather than better. If you follow the diet strictly for the four weeks and still have symptoms then seek professional help.

Any further restrictions on diet or eliminating actual foods should be done under proper supervision by an appropriate professional. (The most common offenders are milk, wheat, eggs, yeast, citrus, tomato and peanuts).

Before consulting a health professional about food or environmental related illness check what their qualifications are in environmental illness specifically and their level of experience.

Allergy/sensitivity has unfortunately become rather 'trendy'. There are a large number of various health professionals now 'dabbling' in allergy with only superficial knowledge and experience.

The AAA (Allergy Association of Australia, PO Box 298, Ringwood, Victoria, 3134) have a list of practitioners with suitable qualifications and experience.

Patients with serious problems will find these suggestions are a useful first step but may require further dietary restrictions and guidance.

## Restrictions

No— sugars added to food or hidden in processed foods. Words ending in '-ose' indicate a sugar: maltose, sucrose, fructose, lactose, glucose, etc. Sugars occurring naturally in foods, eg: fructose in whole fruit are not restricted.

No— added salt

No— chocolate

No— tea or coffee (not even decaffeinated). Use herbal teas or Chinese green tea

No— added sweeteners, flavourings, colourings, or preservatives (even if described as 'natural')

No— commercially frozen or canned foods except well-drained canned fish (tuna, sardines, salmon, mackerel), tinned fruits in their own juice, tinned cooked dried beans (butter beans, kidney beans, etc.) which have been well washed and drained.

No— more than three cups of fresh fruit per day. Fruit juices should be fresh not reconstituted and drunk diluted with water: one part juice to two parts water. A glass of diluted fruit juice counts as one serve of fruit for the day.

No— alcohol

Avoid cigarette smoke. If you are a regular smoker do not attempt to give up until you have been on the diet for at least four weeks but keep a record of the number of cigarettes smoked per day.

## Recommendations

### Diet

Eat whole foods: wholemeal wheat bread, wholemeal rye, wholemeal pasta, brown rice, buckwheat kernels, legumes (soybeans, lentils, kidney beans, etc.) nuts, pumpkin and sunflower seeds, sprouted seeds and beans (alfalfa, munga, etc.).

Any fresh fruit or vegetable. No dried fruit except naturally dried fruit. Fresh meat, particularly fish. Try and reduce red meat to not more than twice weekly and remove all visible fat and skin.

Eat three small main meals and three snacks between meals per day. This helps to stabilise blood glucose levels and increase metabolic rate.

Drink at least eight glasses of water per day as drinks, soups, juices, etc. Water must be filtered or use natural mineral water.

Try to eat a large variety of foods and do not eat a particular food every day, eg: wheat bread. Aim to eat a particular food on not more than two or three days per week.

Steam and grill food where possible and avoid fried foods.

Use vegetable oils (olive oil is best) rather than animal oils or fats.

Avoid yeast or yeast products where possible (Vegemite, etc.) and avoid pickled or cured foods (processed meats, ham, bacon, chutneys, pickled onions, etc.).

Restrict sweeteners to one teaspoon of maple syrup or honey per day.

*Read labels on food packaging so that you know what you are eating.*

**Exercise**

The importance of exercise in improving the functioning of the immune system and cardiovascular system cannot be overestimated.

If you are not doing regular exercise then it is extremely important that you start an exercise programme at the same time as changing your diet. Nearly all people following this diet (so long as they do not over-indulge in nuts or meat) lose excess weight. In order not to lose lean body tissue rather than fat tissue it is vital that exercise is done daily. Exercise also increases the metabolic rate which helps to maintain weight loss.

If you are overweight, unfit and don't do regular exercise check with your doctor before starting any exercise programme. Two cheap and very effective ways of exercising are brisk walking for half an hour per day or following the XBX Programme for women or the 5BX Programme for men which take only ten minutes per day (*Physical Fitness*, Penguin).

## Well what else can I eat?

When trying to increase variety into the diet people often panic. Although there is a bewildering array of 'alternative and health foods' now available, it is often not very obvious what you do with them. Health food shops stock and can provide information on appropriate alternative foods. They are usually extremely obliging at tracking down particular products that may be required.

This section gives a few hints on alternatives and increasing variety in accordance with the general dietary guidelines.

With all packaged foods read labels *very* carefully as the name of the product can be misleading.

### Milk and Dairy Foods

Cows milk can be substituted with a soy milk or coconut milk. Goats milk is worth trying but often still causes sensitivity symptoms.

Try fruit juice or pureed fruit and nuts on cereals.

The most palatable soy milk I have tasted, which even makes lovely sauces, is a fresh soy milk called Excel which is available in supermarkets in NSW but can be difficult to get elsewhere. Start making demands for it at supermarkets and I'm sure it will become freely available!

Eggs can be substituted satisfactorily in recipes by 'Orgran Egg Replacer'.

Butter can be substituted by non-dairy margarines (Sundew, Nuttelex) or in cooking with vegetable oil. Olive oils are best. If you find the taste too strong try Bertolli Light Olive Oil.

**Meat**

Since chemical residues tend to be stored in fat all meat should be trimmed of as much visible fat and skin as possible and grilled or roasted on a rack.

Try reducing the overall consumption of meat although this can be very difficult if there are major grain and milk sensitivities.

Try and obtain genuine free range poultry. Fresh fish is best but canned sardines, tuna and salmon are also good. Remember to rinse off any brine.

Occasionally, if available, try quail, venison, turkey to vary the type of meat eaten. Local butchers can also be extremely helpful by making up gluten free and chemically free sausages with alternative meats to beef.

**Grains**

There is now a large range of alternative grain products on the market. Breads: rye, one hundred percent sour dough breads (with no added gluten) have a fine texture and even children find it easy to switch to these non-wheat breads ('Wuppertaler'—plain sour dough, loaves, rolls, flat bread, fruit bread), Ri-ota, Wupperbrot.

**Pastas**

Orgran corn, buckwheat, barley and spinach, rice and millet, rye, legume pastas are now freely available from health food stores.

These can be served with simple tomato-based sauces or if tomatoes are a problem: olive oil and garlic, grated vegetables and herbs, kidney beans, etc. tossed through the pasta while it is hot.

**Dry Biscuits**

Russell's Rice Cakes ('polystyrene biscuits' some patients call them!) can be used for spreads or crumbed to use instead of breadcrumbs. Kasha (buckwheat) Crispbread, Rice Cruskits, Rye Cruskits, Edwards and Son Rice Snaps.

**Pancakes**

Frankly I find most non-wheat pancakes quite inedible—a bit like chewing rubber! But either of the batters below made very thin and cooked as 'crepes' in a large pan make an extremely satisfactory alternative. Pour a little batter into a lavishly oiled (forget Pritikin!) pan and spread out to the edges with a spatula. Turn once then serve with pureed fruit or one of the sugarless jams or marmalades.

BUCKWHEAT BATTER

1 cup buckwheat flour
½ teaspoon bicarb. soda or baking powder
Whisk with enough water to make a thin batter

THREE FLOURS BATTER

⅓ cup dried pea flour
⅓ cup rice flour
⅓ cup millet meal
½ teaspoon bicarb. soda or baking powder
Whisk with enough water to make a thin batter

**Breakfast Cereals**

Puffed single grains, eg: rice, millet, buckwheat, corn flakes, weeties, porridge.

Avoid mueslis which are a combination of several grains.

A breakfast alternative is mashed banana mixed with raw rolled oats, nuts and naturally dried fruit.

Porridge without milk can be rather disappointing but the natural creaminess of oats can be used to make a porridge more like 'gruel' which is very creamy and especially good with maple syrup or honey.

Creamy porridge: use rolled oats and substitute water for the milk. While porridge is cooking beat it with a handbeater or, alternatively, put the raw oats in a food processor until they have a fine texture before cooking. Add water to achieve the desired consistency.

### Fruit and Bran Muffins

Some people who have trouble with a grain or grains find they can tolerate the bran only of the grain. These brans can be milled further in a food processor to make quite acceptable 'flours' to use in cooking. Any bran will do but I've found rice and oat brans best.

2 very ripe bananas or 1 cup other fruit (grated apple, apricots etc.)
2½ cups rice bran *or* oat bran
1 rounded tablespoon baking powder *or* bicarb. soda
¼ cup brown sugar or 1 tablespoon honey
1½ cups water
2 tablespoons vegetable oil

Heat oven to 220°C and put gem irons or muffin pans in oven to heat. Put bran in food processor for five minutes, add oil, baking powder and bananas/fruit and process. Add honey and water, process to a smooth batter.

Take gem irons or muffin irons out of oven and brush with oil or use patty pans. Pour in batter. Bake 10–15 mins. Remove from oven and turn out onto rack. Delicious eaten hot, quite edible cold.

For orange flavoured muffins substitute water with fresh orange juice and grated rind of two oranges.

Two easy non-wheat lunch box treats are as follows:

OAT BISCUITS

2 tablespoons oil or margarine
2 tablespoons honey

Boil together. Add enough rolled oats to make a stiff sticky mixture. Press into a slab tin. Bake at 375°C for ten minutes or just brown at the edges. Place in the fridge until very cold and cut into squares.

RICE, CORN OR BUCKWHEAT CRUNCH

1 tablespoon honey
1 tablespoon oil or margarine

Boil together for three minutes stirring continuously. Add four cups of either cornflakes *or* rice bubbles *or* puffed buckwheat.

Quickly fill patty pans with mixture and bake in a moderate oven for three to four minutes or until just changing colour. Allow to cool.

**Spreads, Dips and Chutneys**

There are now a range of sugar free 'jams' and marmalades available—Spiral Foods, Pro Soba, Wright Farm, Natures Own, Glen Ewin. Avoid 'diet' foods as they are usually loaded with additives.

Maple syrup, nut spreads, fresh fruit purees (eg: apricot), date spreads, avocado dip. Hummus is an excellent source of calcium as well as being a useful spread or dip. Make your own or use 'instant humus', available in health food stores.

Nut butters, eg: cashew, almond, are expensive but if you have major sensitivities may be necessary.

**Fruits**

There really are more fruits than apples, oranges and bananas. Try (according to your bank balance!) avocados, kiwifruit, passionfruit, watermelon, canteloupe, pineapple, tamarillo, guavas, mango, etc.

For those wanting a 'filling' food a fruit pudding can be made to eat hot or cold from tapioca, fruit juice or water and pureed fruit.

FRUIT PUDDING

4 tablespoons tapioca
1 cup water or fruit juice
2 cups pureed fruit (apricots, or peaches, or canteloupe, or mango, or passionfruit).

Stir the tapioca in the liquid on low heat until tapioca is clear. Stir in pureed fruit and eat hot or allow to set in the fridge. Out of season canned fruits in their own juice (no sugar) can be a satisfactory alternative to fresh fruit.

**Vegetables**

Similarly, there are more vegetables than potatoes, carrots and peas.

Try sweet potato (yummy roasted), celeriac, taro, parsnips (better roasted), butternut pumpkin, broad beans, green beans, cos lettuce, zucchini, marrow, sprouted seeds and beans.

Childen often like vegetables raw or cooked and chilled with dressing or a dip better than hot vegetables.

To increase variety and decrease the number of times a vegetable is eaten try having more of one or two vegetables each night rather than a small amount each of three to four vegetables.

Most vegetables can be put into mixed soups or pureed as single vegetable soups, eg: zucchini, pumpkin, carrot, sweet potato, onion, broccoli, cauliflower. Children often find a pureed soup more acceptable than 'soup with bits of things'.

Vegetable patties can be made by using one vegetable mashed as a base, eg: potato, sweet potato or pumpkin and adding chopped or grated onion, celery, carrot, broccoli, cauliflower. Roll in crushed rice biscuits or rice bubbles and fry.

Vegetable pancakes can be made by grating vegetables (single or mixed) and frying spoonfuls of mixture in a pan.

**Legumes**

Legumes are an excellent source of fibre and protein.

Tinned beans (three bean mix, kidney beans, etc.) are convenient and generally acceptable if they are washed very well and soaked for a few minutes.

They can be eaten alone, in salads or added to soups.

BEAN SALAD

1 can Three bean mix (washed thoroughly)
1 cup chopped celery
1 cup corn kernels
½ cup spring onions
1 red capsicum chopped

Toss with lemon juice and olive oil. Add black pepper to taste.

The first few weeks modifying your diet (and particularly your family's!) can be hell but most people find that within two to three weeks the dietary guidelines are not particularly hard to follow.

But remember good eating should lead to good living—it should not become an almost religious obsession.

The following cookbooks are excellent for widening variety and have alternative recipes eliminating foods to which people are commonly sensitive:

*Australian Food Allergy Cookbook* by Janelle Chant, Sally Lee and Jenny Murrowood, Sun Books.

*Comprehensive Allergy Cookbook* by Kate Bellamy, Fontana/Collins.

*Recipes to the Rescue* by Lindy Kingsmill, Suzanne Morrow, Pam Bonner, Greenhouse.

# CHAPTER NINE

# Coping with Yourself and Your Children

An overwhelming feeling of patients with sensitivities (children and adults) is that their life is out of their physical and emotional control.

These patients suffer enormous stress. Sensitivities interfere with a person's ability to adapt physically and emotionally to his or her environment. Stress occurs when the physical and emotional 'stressors' on a person exceed that person's ability to adapt.

This stress weakens the immune system further, creating a vicious circle which can be extraordinarily difficult to break.

If there has been a long period of misdiagnosis of their symptoms, patients may feel they have to prove they are sick to family, friends, and government agencies pending sickness benefits or compensation. This leads to a great deal of negative emotion (eg: anger) and anguish which can exhaust their limited resources and stop them getting better even when they are effectively minimising their exposures. They can burn up so much energy proving they are sick and fighting bureaucracies that there is little left to fight the illness itself.

It is crucial that a reliable diagnosis of food/chemical sensitivity is made as quickly as possible before the anger and anguish take over.

As with all other illnesses which go through an acute phase to become chronic, there is a real danger that patients will start to receive emotional payoffs from the illness. In fact, patients who have been ill for a long time can find that peers and families prefer them ill. Mind you, if a chronic illness means your life is hell maybe you need a few payoffs!

Emotional payoffs from being ill are a significant problem when they stop the patient from getting well or are used to manipulate other people.

The adjustments that sensitivity patients need to make can seem overwhelmingly difficult at first. Denial is a common reaction, as with other serious illness. Denial can be an extremely positive strategy in some types of illness and for particular patients, but with true sensitivities denial just makes things worse in the long term. The body's immune system just can't cope or get over sensitivities if the patient blindly continues exposing him or herself to allergens regardless of symptoms.

Once diagnosed, patients and their families need to get over their anger as quickly as possible (with professional help if necessary) in order to get on with dealing with the problem. Life throws a series of uncontrollable events at all of us. Anguish is something we create ourselves when we fight against these events.

Most ill people at some stage say 'it isn't fair'. Face facts: the idea of fairness is a fantasy, a fairy story we give our children to make them less self-centered, more sociable and easier for us to live with.

Fairness is a lovely ideal but it is not a reality. What is fair in the world? In Australia most of us have enough to eat and a roof over our heads. In many other countries most people are hungry with no shelter.

The same goes for illness. Some people's sensitivities are serious and others are negligible. What really makes sensitivity patients scream 'it isn't fair' is that it all appears so preventable—and that's a social issue bigger than any individual.

Patients must separate what they can do in terms of lobbying the social issue and what they can do for themselves and their family.

In our society the patient's first responsibility must be to themselves and their family. If there is any time left over then he or she may choose to get involved with others in lobbying the social issues or helping other patients.

Once the patient accepts the problem, they need to write a list of what recommendations have been made and their priorities. Accurate information may have to come from a number of disiplines—not just psychology or medicine.

Once a patient has a list of recommendations and their priorities, they need to look at what is possible in their circumstances. Many of the decisions will need to be made after discussion with the rest of the family. The discussion will need to be totally honest.

Once decisions are made, accept them and get on with carrying them out. As many patients have a great deal of difficulty with even simple decision making, professional help from a counsellor may be time and cost saving long term. Even if some decisions turn out in hindsight not to have been the best possible the point is that they seemed the best at the time.

Patients can't afford to waste time trying to prove their illness. Even if engaged in a medico-legal claim they need to make sure the professionals involved fight for them properly. They can't afford the energy to get too involved themselves. Assertiveness training can be a powerful psychological weapon for these patients as it gives them the confidence to accept themselves and their limitations.

The immune system and mind are intimately connected and in constant two-way communication with each other. Some of the best techniques for minimising the stress reaction to the illness and decreasing the degree of sensitivity are psychological.

Cognitive (thinking) techniques can help keep emotional responses due to sensitivities under control. Generally speaking, what you tell yourself about a situation controls your emotional response, ie: emotions come from your thinking not the situation.

For instance, if you greet someone you know well in the street and they ignore you, you might say to yourself: 'How dare they ignore me! What have I done to deserve this sort of treatment?' This sort of reaction results in anger, hurt and feelings of rejection. Alternatively you might have said to yourself: 'His mind must have been elsewhere' resulting in a neutral emotional response.

Similarly, sensitivity patients who experience rapid mood changes which seem to 'wash' over them for no apparent reason can say to themselves: 'I feel anxious and tearful for no reason. I must be having a breakdown'. This results in feelings of fear, isolation and further anxiety. Or they can say to themselves: 'Today I seem to be having a bad day but I know it will pass as it has before. I'll do some meditation which I know will help'. This results in positive feelings and allows the patient to adopt a helpful strategy.

With children, these cognitive strategies are extremely important to help the child see themselves as having some control over their life and stop the child using their sensitivities as an excuse for being thoroughly obnoxious.

Even if a child has severe behavioural disturbances with reactions they need to be given positive strategies for dealing with themselves when they have the symptoms. For instance, just because egg turns a child into a pint-size Attilla the Hun doesn't mean to say he is excused from responsibility for bashing the dog with a baseball bat after unwittingly consuming egg in a biscuit.

The child must be taught to recognise symptoms developing before they are out of hand and how to take appropriate steps to minimise the effects.

For instance, by taking Buffered C, prescribed homeopathic sublingual drops or by removing himself to his cubby house or room on his own for a while until symptoms subside.

One of my small patients became very good at recognising the cranky, aggressive and panicky feelings he developed when exposed to diesel fumes. When asked about what he did when he felt these feelings coming on he told me he would find his mother to give him the drops 'that take the bad out of me'.

A punching bag in the garden is also a wonderful way for aggressive children (and adults) to vent frustration and anger.

The behaviour of sensitive children can be so socially undesirable that they receive overwhelmingly negative and extremely little positive feedback about themselves. They not only lose self-esteem but often they never get a chance to develop any in the first place! The sobbing plea of one five-year-old after appalling behaviour says it all: 'I'm not a *bad* boy. It's just that the good boy gets lost'.

Cognitive strategies can help build self-esteem. A child who finds themself in rages for no reason is just as frightened as the others nearby and can be quite mortified afterwards by their lack of control.

The child who is extremely anxious and cannot cope easily with separation still has to go to school and learn to deal with the feelings. 'When I leave Mum I get an uncomfortable feeling inside but I know I will get used to leaving Mum and then the feelings will go away. Most kids feel like this sometimes'. This is a much more constructive thinking process which will diminish natural anxiety. Compare it to: 'Mum's going to leave me. I'm scared stiff, I can't stand it. Nobody else feels like this'.

Discuss not only how the child feels but point out to them the words they are telling themselves about the situation. Then substitute better things the child can tell themself and get them to practise out loud. Explain how they can be unhappy or happy about any situation depending on what they tell him or herself. 'My birthday's next week and I'm getting a bicycle. Won't that be great?' Compare this with: 'My birthday's next week and I'm getting a bicycle but not the colour I want and I'm not allowed to have a party. Poor me'.

Children and adults with sensitivities also benefit from any psychological techniques which reduce emotional stress and its consequent effect on the immune system, eg: deep relaxation, especially if combined with biofeedback, guided imagery, hypnotherapy or psychoimmunological subliminal tapes. These techniques need to be taught by a clinical psychologist. Transcendental meditation, yoga, tai chi, and martial arts can also be excellent methods for improving immune function by reducing emotional stress. Find a technique that suits you.

# Behavioural management of children and adolescents

## Accurate diagnosis

It is crucial that an accurate diagnosis is made of any sensitivities as early as possible and exposure to them minimised.

The following suggestions will not be effective long term unless priority is given to any physical problems.

## Acceptance

No matter how unfair it may seem these children have to be helped to find ways of dealing with their sensitivities in a physically hostile world. As soon as the diagnosis is made and children are able to start manipulating their world verbally or non-verbally, they must be given as much responsibility for their health and the consequences of their behaviour as possible.

If children are not made to realise this is mainly their problem and their responsibility they tend to start blaming parents, teachers and the world at large for everything that is wrong in their lives. Special diets can be seen as something for others' benefit rather than the child's. When the child says, 'It isn't fair', agree—it isn't. But that's just the way it is. Don't allow children to fight the situation and create a nightmare of anguish for them and you. Force them to accept the problem and help them deal with it. Parents who are anguished because they can't accept their own or their children's sensitivities themselves will never get their children to accept them either. Such families are riddled with anger, guilt and ill health. They oscillate between outright denial—neglecting to minimise their exposures and becoming ill—or obsessive adherence to details without looking at the major problems—hanging newspapers and books on the clothesline to air before reading but continuing to smoke.

Such parents often demand strict adherence by others (particularly schools or workmates) to stop polluting the air but make only minor changes in their own lifestyle. If parents find they cannot accept the situation and deal with it constructively they should seek professional help.

## Balancing physical and emotional needs

Just as with adults, children need to work out what is possible and what is ideal. For the sake of their social and emotional development they may be forced to put up with some degree of symptoms.

Your child may feel that developing a rash and not sleeping very well is a small price to pay for being able to eat like everyone else at a birthday party. (You can make it easier by making sure the child has a substantial snack of permissable food before going to the party so he or she is less likely to fill up on junk food.) Of course, children who have serious reactions can be helped by subtly making sure that permissable foods which are attractive to other children as well are also available.

Point out to a child that other children may have glasses, caliper, hearing aid, etc. so that the child sees his or her own problems in perspective. Having sensitivities is tough but so is being blind.

## Sibling rivalry and role playing

If a child is the only child in the family to have allergies/ sensitivities there is a real risk that the child can be given or take on the role of being the 'problem' in the family (or at school).

Other children can play on the situation beautifully and either set the child up knowing they have a 'short fuse', tease them, or be extremely 'good' themselves in order to show the child up even more. This is no good for either child. The child with sensitivities soon gives up trying and fulfills the 'bad' role they are given. The 'good' child won't allow themself human frailties.

Acknowledge that it may be tougher for the child with sensitivities to control their behaviour but they still have to take responsibility for it and find strategies for avoiding conflict. The behaviour is ultimately their responsibility, not other people's.

Show your child they have a choice. If other children are teasing or being nasty, let your child know *they don't have to* get upset or react. To react or not is their decision. 'Sensitive' children are often very good at shifting blame: 'You made me upset'.

## A structured routine

Since these children may feel their bodies and minds are out of control, external structure in their routine can reduce their anxiety and give them some feeling of security. Since their auditory memory, idea of time and consequences can be poor, a chart of their routine (in pictures if necessary) can give a visual representation of the order of daily and weekly activities.

eg: Before school
Get up and make bed
Wash
Dress
Pack bag and lunch
Check which day it is
Breakfast
Coat and bag
School

WEEKLY ROUTINE

| Mon | Tues | Wed | Thurs | Fri | Sat | Sun |
|---|---|---|---|---|---|---|
| School | School | School | School | School | | |
| | Music (take recorder) | Sport (take sports shoes) | Tennis (take racquet) | | Football | |
| Swimming (take bathers) | | | | Friend from school | | |
| | | | Cubs (take uniform) | | | |

Keep a strict routine for meal times, bed times and after school, eg: play, dinner, bath, story, bed.

## Methods of disipline

As discussed earlier these children can be totally inconsequential and live only for the present. This can make them very difficult to discipline. However, difficult to discipline isn't an excuse not to discipline.

## 1. 'Time-out'

This can be a very effective technique to use with children who are reacting. Rather than punish the reacting child, it is better to remove the child from the situation they cannot cope with for a few minutes, giving them (and the parents) a chance to regain control.

To be effective, 'time-out' demands that the parent remains calm, totally in control and firm. The child is told that they are being isolated so that they have a chance to 'feel better' or behave as is appropriate to the situation, eg: play with another child rather than bit him.

Before a misdemeanor occurs, explain to the child that whenever they do X, they will be isolated in some way for five minutes, to give them a chance to feel better.

To isolate a child, choose a 'neutral' place that is safe but uninteresting. A bathroom with locked cupboards, a hallway or even the garden if the child is claustrophobic. Time-out is not punishment, but a neutral consequence of unacceptable behaviour to give the child a chance to regain control. NEVER isolate a child in a place that is punitive or frightening, eg: a cupboard or dark room.

Immediately the child misbehaves, don't berate, scream or abuse. Calmly and firmly take the child and put them where they are to be isolated. Tell the child matter-of-factly what they did wrong and that they can come out in five minutes. The first few times, the child may kick, scream or become quite hysterical (you may have to hold the door shut). STAY CALM! At the end of the five minutes, open the door and walk away. *Don't* stand there, glaring at him or her, creating a confrontation with: 'Are you going to be good now?' or 'Say you're sorry'.

This creates a confrontation which the child will want to win to save face. Simply open the door and busy yourself with some other task well away from the child.

Act as if the behaviour is not your responsibility. If the child repeats the behaviour, immediately repeat the time-out procedure.

Once the child realises that you are not getting upset, and that they are the only loser, they will quickly respond.

Don't work on more than one aberrant behaviour at any one time (otherwise the child will always be in time-out!), and decide priorities on which behaviour you choose to work on, eg: biting may be your top priority. Once one misbehaviour is controlled, start on another.

Usually, just when you feel that you have a behaviour controlled, they seem to regress worse than ever. This also occurs when training animals. Don't despair, but persevere as before. It is usually a sort of 'last fling' before the behaviour is permanently changed.

**2. Logical consequences**

Since these children tend to be inconsequential, long-term consequences for their behaviour are usually meaningless. However, the most effective way of gaining cooperation from children with sensitivities is to work on *immediate logical* consequences of their behaviour.

This is also one of the rare management techniques that works just as well with teenagers as with small children! Many theories work very well while the child is smaller than the adult, but are hopeless once the child becomes the same size or bigger.

All discipline techniques work best for longer periods, if started when the child is very young rather than when a sixteen-year-old is out of control.

Basically, cooperation is gained not by a system of punishment or denial, but by the child having to accept logical consequences of his or her behaviour. With this approach, the difficult, contrary and aggressive behaviour of a child with sensitivities can be made his or her direct responsibility, thus avoiding opportunities for the child to blame others for their behaviour: 'You made me upset, so I hit the dog!' or 'If you hadn't been cross with me, I wouldn't have forgotten to feed the dog.'

Rather than nag until something is done, give the child a logical consequence if he or she does not complete the task. The consequences are related to the principle that all members of a family have obligations to the successful running of the family unit: parents are bread-winners, shoppers, cooks, housekeepers. Children do homework and chores appropriate to their age, feed and dress themselves, tidy their rooms, bathe themselves and generally behave in a socially acceptable manner. In return, family members receive benefits and privileges from the efforts of the family as a whole: shelter, food, entertainment, hobby material, clothes, transport, education, pocket money, etc.

A family member can only expect the benefits of being in a family if he or she pulls his weight, eg: if morning chores are not done, and if the child is not dressed and ready for school, then he or she gets no breakfast or anything else until they are done. No access to the TV until other commitments are fulfilled. If a child wants to behave like a baby (refusing to dress themself when you know they can), then that is OK, but they will then be treated like a baby and will have to have a morning and afternoon nap like babies do. Alternatively, babies don't watch TV.

The trick is to let the child think that you are ambivalent to which option they choose—cooperation or consequence—and the choice is entirely up to the child.

Once there is no longer a battle of wills involved between you and the child, and he or she is the loser, it becomes easier to just do what is required. The choice to cooperate is seen as the sensible and logical option as the consequences are immediate.

Some parents and professionals are horrified that such

demands be put on children or that it ever be suggested that food be denied until a responsibility is met. But that is what life is all about—you don't work, you don't eat. And the sooner children realise that life is not a free ride, the happier and more responsible they will be. Many children are effectively 'on the dole' from age three receiving full benefits without any work.

Realistic discipline can also be given by seeing pocket money as separate from earned money. Pocket money is a token amount received because you are a member of the family and enjoy the benefits. This money is never 'fined' and therefore encourages a sense of independence and the value of money. Earned money is exactly that—earned for extra jobs outside the home or around the home. For really serious misdemeanors, this earned money may be realistically 'fined', just as adults can be for breaches of the law. Fines should always be an absolute last resort.

The child who is firmly entrenched in a habit of not cooperating as a 'matter of principle' can be made more cooperative by giving him or her a genuine choice with no conflicting messages. If you want something done, don't give conflicting messages by saying: 'Would you mind doing . . .' if you really mean 'Do it now!' To gain cooperation, genuinely request things to be done, with a genuine option not to comply. The first requests will probably be met with a sharp 'no' or 'later'. If you accept that as OK, then requests are no longer seen as a battle of wills, but as an opportunity to genuinely do something for you. Even the most hardened children like approval and respect. When you genuinely make a request, the child feels that he or she has your respect. When trying this initially, it helps to stack the cards in your favour by making requests that don't really matter to you. If you can convey that your request has a genuine option to say no without 'reprisals' then, very soon, requests will be met with a cheery 'yes'. Don't over-react when this happens or applaud loudly the child's sudden change of tune or he or she may panic and decide to revert to contrariness. Simply acknowledge the 'yes' with a matter-of-fact 'thank you' and don't make an issue of their new found maturity.

With all suggestions about managing children and our attempts to turn them into social beings, it should be remembered that children, to a large degree, seem to grow up in spite of us parents, rather than because of us! These are suggestions, and should be considered in the light of your own particular child and your own particular circumstances.

If you feel the situation is out of control, or you feel out of control, then seek professional help immediately! If pushed far enough, all of us are capable of abusing children and, sadly, child abuse is a common occurrence in children with sensitivities. Similarly, the aggressive child can become a highly dangerous teenager and adult, terrorising his or her parents and siblings. Parental and sibling abuse is a hidden and insidious problem which is rarely recognised.

Better still, don't wait for a situation to be out of control. Seek help when you feel instinctively that something is wrong, and remember, children are supposed to be enjoyed not endured.

### 3. Smacking

For young children who still have poor language and reasoning abilities, a *single* sharp immediate smack on the back of the legs may be the most effective means of getting the message across that the behaviour is unacceptable. Here the aim is not to hurt the child or relieve tension in the parent but to give information effectively and quickly, eg: toddlers who keep running on to the road, touching electrical equipment, etc.

For children with sensitivities who are inconsequential and therefore fail to understand danger in such situations, this can be your only option in order to protect your child.

**4. Consistency**

Before deciding a rule of behaviour ask yourself: 'Is it really important?', eg: cleanliness is important, but is tidiness really necessary?

Reduce rules of behaviour to the absolutely essential, and then be consistent in making sure they are carried out.

**5. Confusion**

When reacting, children with sensitivities may appear dazed and confused. At those times, they will have difficulty in understanding instructions and remembering to carry them out. They will also become good at 'playing' at reacting in order to avoid unpleasant tasks. This occasional 'play acting' can leave parents and teachers extremely confused, frustrated and angry if they feel they are being duped.

Parents and teachers dealing with these children need to rely a great deal on instinct as particular situations arise.

If you get the feeling that the child is 'trying you out', you are probably right and extra pressure to complete the task is probably warranted. But, if the child appears genuinely anxious about being confused and looks at you blankly, then it would be more appropriate to accept that the child is reacting and take appropriate measures.

You must remember that children with sensitivities may well be able, with enormous effort, to complete tasks. However, the effort necessary means that they can tire very easily. Performance may be fine to start with, but they deteriorate quickly during a lesson. The rewards and self-satisfaction they get from completing a task may be meagre compared to the effort that has to be made. Hence, they tend to give up and avoid academic work.

# Specific problems

## Self-esteem

Since the effort required may be out of all proportion to the rewards gained in both social skills and schoolwork, and since they often feel 'out of control', children with sensitivities have little self-esteem.

It can be very difficult to build self-esteem in a child who sees him or herself as constantly doing the wrong thing and being continually reprimanded.

Adults need to be extremely careful about what they say in front of the child to other parents, relatives, teachers and health professionals. Insist that discussions about the child with health professionals occur in the absence of the child. 'He is driving me up the wall' should only be said to a health professional in private.

Try and find qualities and interests in the child unique to that child and which do not put him or her in direct competition with his or her siblings. Talk about these qualities to other parents and professionals in the child's hearing. 'Jack has such lovely curly hair and such big brown eyes'. Or, 'Jack is so responsible with his diet. He is more sensible than some adults in what he eats.' Or, 'Jack is becoming a great help in the kitchen'.

Find positive roles for the child in the family which also gives you a chance to talk to them, not at them. Helping to get dinner can be a chance to talk.

Recognise the extra effort involved to carry out tasks and praise the effort not the result. 'I really admire how you finished that project. I could see that you kept going, even though you were so tired.' Or, 'It's great the way you kept your cool when Tommy smashed your bike. That must have been hard.'

Use positive labels to influence the child's perception of themselves. If you call a child responsible or sensible often enough (even if initially, they aren't), then that is what the child tends to become. Similarly, the more you call the child a nuisance, lazy or a slob, the more they live up to that label too.

Positive labels are especially powerful when uttered by significant others in the child's life, such as a favourite aunt, or by authority figures such as the school principal, teacher or health professional. We all respond to praise and recognition and children with sensitivities are no different.

Find excuses occasionally to go out with the child on his or her own without other siblings. If necessary, take the child out of school for a day to visit the dentist, buy clothes and have lunch together. This gives parents a unique opportunity to get to know and keep in touch with the child as an individual, and not just as 'one of the children'. This is just as important for the siblings of a child with sensitivities.

## Shyness

Children with sensitivities are often extremely timid and have difficulty adjusting to any new situation or different people. Just as they tend to over-react physically, so also, they tend to over-react emotionally.

If these children are allowed to escape facing new situations and people, they can end up with serious social and emotional handicaps by the time they are teenagers. This can develop into serious depression. Others may learn to use their ill health to avoid social or family obligations.

Timid children need to be gently encouraged to tackle new and different situations while they are young, and to tackle them in realistic steps.

When your child complains of 'scary feelings inside', point out that everybody has those feelings in particular situations, and that they are caused by the body getting ready to do its best. The feelings are like being excited about Christmas. Whether they are 'scary' or 'exciting', depends on what the child decides to tell him or herself about the situation: 'I've got those strange feelings again, because I'm scared of going to the birthday party on my own' or 'I've got those strange feelings again, because I'm excited about the birthday party and the good time I'm going to have'.

Be understanding and help the child to gradually settle into new surroundings with increasing absences from Mum and Dad. Visit the home of their friends from school and get to know their parents. If your child sees you are comfortable with their friends and their families, they will also be comfortable. Reassure the child that you will never leave them in the care of someone you do not trust to look after them properly. Spend time helping out at the school with reading, etc. If the child sees you are happy, they will be to. If you drop the child at the gate and flee, avoiding staff and other parents, they won't want to stay either. Many parents, particularly single parents, don't have the choice of easing their child into school, creches etc, and in these cases, strong messages to the child that they can and will cope with their feelings if they choose to, can be the only real option. In this situation, parents must be very sure of who the child is to stay with and remain calm and firm as the child screams and clings pleading not to be left.

Tell your child firmly that everyone feels a bit strange with different people, but it is up to them whether they get upset or not. This gives the child some feelings of control and with this comes confidence to adapt. 'You don't have to get upset'. *Never deny* the child's feelings, but show the child they have a choice of how they react to them.

Many children are quite happy to have children visit their home and to have their own birthday party, but resist all attempts to induce them to visit their friends on their own.

It is not fair to the other child if your child always wants the friendship on their own terms.

Explain that friendships are two-way and require effort by both people. The first couple of times, go with the child for a short visit. When your child is in the middle of a good game with their friend, say that you have to go home to clean his or her room, and ask if your child would like to stay a bit longer. Gradually, as confidence grows, the child's desire to complete the game will override wanting to go home with you to clean up their room!

With parties, it is hardly fair if your child expects ten friends and ten presents and continually refuses to go to any of their friends' parties. Point out that parties are only successful when everyone decides to enjoy themselves and join in, and just as a host has responsibilities, so does a guest who is invited.

Again, visit their friend's house before the party, so that your child can 'check it out'. Sometimes, it is easier if another parent, whom they know well, and whose child is also going to the party, picks your child up from home. In the way, the excitement and familiarity of the other child overrides any anxiety.

If a child continually and absolutely refuses to make any attempt to attend a party, even with one of their own parents staying, calmly point out that it's OK to make this decision, but your child cannot then expect to have a party until they are big enough to at least try to be a guest.

Insist that, as a guest, your child must at least take the birthday child a present. Once they are actually at the party, Mum can often leave without too much trouble. Indicate that your child can decide to enjoy themself, or decide to get upset. It's up to them, not you, the parent. Once a child is confronted with the fact that their mother cannot control their feelings, there ceases to be much point in performing.

This approach may seem at odds with what was said earlier about these children's emotions being affected by their sensitivities. However, in the 'real world' the child can't afford to feel that they are some helpless victim, but must be given ways of taking control. Certainly, it might be harder, and this should be recognised, but ultimately, with support and encouragement, the child has to toughen up if they are to survive emotionally and socially.

The child with sensitivities who is also emotionally sensitive, can use their sensitiveness positively to develop a maturity and empathy beyond their years. Used constructively, emotional sensitivity can be the child's biggest asset. Uncontrolled, it can destroy him or her. You must show the child it is his or her decision.

## Siblings

For siblings without sensitivities it can be extremely difficult living with a child whose behaviour and health is so unpredictable and who often receives a great deal of attention (even if negative) from their parents.

The plight of these children also needs recognition. If at all possible, give other siblings their own room or place in the house where they can get away and their privacy is totally respected.

Aknowledge to these children that what they have to put up with can be frustrating and upsetting. If the children can see you recognise their side of the story you have a good chance of them cooperating with you. Honest communication, explanation of the sensitivities and empathy with their predicament as well as time alone with each sibling can overcome any problems very well and lead to much greater maturity and responsibility in the siblings.

As mentioned earlier, it is vital that siblings are not allowed to use a child with sensitivities as a scapegoat and that siblings are also free to be 'human'.

## Aggression

Aggression can be a very serious problem with these children and adolescents. Aggression due exclusively to sensitivities is entirely spontaneous and not at all premeditated. However, secondary psychological factors can begin to operate very early with agressive children and this combined with their anger and irritability can turn them into rather 'nasty' individuals.

New theories see agression as 'disinhibition', possibly due to problems in seratonin metabolism in the brain. This is certainly consistent with the various possibilities regarding the mechanism of sensitivity (outlined in Chapter 1). Many of these children bite rather than hit. There is evidence that biproducts of the metabolism of cow's milk can trigger aggressive outbursts. Endless explanations of why aggressive behaviour is not acceptable is generally a waste of time as the child is quite aware after the event that what they did was wrong. The child can be very shocked and upset by their behaviour.

With aggression caused by sensitivities, the situation can be extremely dangerous as the child may not inhibit the severity of this outburst before it is too late.

The usual approach is to isolate a child ('time-out') for a period of five minutes (no more or they will forget why they are being isolated and think it's all your fault!).

If this does not work then professional help should be sought immediately as other children (and adults) must be protected.

## Fighting

Aggression in these children can be extreme, unprovoked and come with no warning. During such episodes, they may seem impervious to pain.

The best option is always 'time-out'. However, since

these children very quickly become scapegoats for other children and are often cunningly set-up, it is often best to give 'time-out' to both children involved—in separate rooms!

This encourages other children to take steps to avoid conflicts and not deliberately provoke an incident.

## Seeking help

There are probably as many effective ways of disciplining children as there are children. There are now countless books written on how and how not to manage children. Unfortunately, many of these textbook techniques fail because the children don't read the books, and therefore tend to break the rules of predicted behaviour! Books on child management (particularly if the child has sensitivities) can leave parents extremely bewildered when the child doesn't behave or respond according to the book! If you are having management problems, and your child's diet is sound and chemical exposure is as minimal as you can make it, then seek expert help from a child psychologist. Even one or two individual sessions can make an enormous difference, as management is discussed in terms of your particular family and child not the mythical average child.

Follow-up sessions in a group setting can be far more rewarding if individual problems are considered first.

If you attend group programmes, eg: Parent Effectiveness Training (PET) or Systematic Training for Effective Parenting (STEP), don't accept them uncritically (remember most have been written by males who have rarely been all day child care givers). Always relate the suggestions made to your particular situations and values. If you are in doubt, have the group leader look at your particular problem in more detail. Choose a leader who is a very experienced practitioner (not an academic with little practical experience) who is also a psychologist with a wider understanding and experience of child management than just that one approach.

## Mobilising resources

Patients coping with their own sensitivities as well as their childrens' are prime candidates for developing the 'screaming heeby-jeebies' (breaking-point) at some time when they least expect it. At these times, it is vital for the emotional and physical well-being of the children that the parents are aware of the community and personal resources available to help them. Better still, they should make use of these resources in order to avoid actually reaching breaking-point.

Women are especially vulnerable as the modern woman in many cases has exchanged her handcuffs (not being allowed to do what she wants to) for a ball and chain (now tired and worn out trying to do everything).

When you are sick, or when your children are sick, you need all the help you can get. Be assertive and ruthless. If you need help, don't ask for it—demand it!

Don't put all your eggs in one basket and wear out one resource—your partner. Spread the load and work out what you can realistically expect from partners, family, friends, psychologist, GP, paediatrician, Citizens Advice Bureau,school, teachers, local councils, family day care, home help, community health centres etc.

Local councils are a good point to start, as their community development officers coordinate an enormous and diverse range of government and voluntary services available in your particular community.

The stress that sensitivities and chronic ill health place on families and particularly the primary caregiver of the children is understandable, but it is inexcusable for parents to need help and not seek it, thus putting their children at risk. It is the responsibility of health professionals and the community in general to empathise with the stress that these people may be under, so that they recognise the signs of families at risk and offer constructive help. If you feel you need help urgently out of business hours, ring 'Lifeline'.

# Summary of suggestions for surviving allergic/sensitive children at home and in the classroom

**Structure and routine**

**Consistency of rules and consequences**

**Discipline**

- 'Time-out' procedure
- Taking the logical consequences of their behaviour
- Negotiation rather than confrontation
- Decide what rules are really important and worth the battle
- Action rather than words, eg: remove a forbidden object but don't lecture and plead

**Instructions**

- Stand directly in front of the child and be sure you have eye contact
- Use short simple sentences only
  Do not give more than one or two instructions at a time
- Speak slowly
- Use visual aids either written or in pictures to aid memory
- If necessary place hands gently on child's shoulders to direct attention

**Responsibility**

- Be understanding of the extra effort required but put responsibility for the consequences of sensitivity reactions firmly on the child

**Self-esteem**

- Build self-esteem by rewarding effort rather than result
- Find 'special' interests which are different from siblings and peers
- Find time to give individual children positive attention
- Discuss options rather than demand obedience to instructions

—Get the child involved in their own health decisions

**For teachers**

—Note the above suggestions and also:

—Discourage parents from asking for daily reports on progress or misdemeanors, etc. Give reports only at usual times

—Gain a written list of all child's known allergies/ sensitivities

—Check classroom for possible problem materials and substitute or remove if at all possible to storerooms with outside ventilation, eg: spirit pens, freshly printed materials, paints, glues, soft plastics, etc.

—Ventilation: make sure the room is properly aired (using fans if necessary every lunchtime and recess)

—Use safe cleaning products only. Steam clean carpets with water only

—Ban smoking, perfumes, hairsprays, etc.

—Check heating systems are working efficiently

—Before buying new equipment or furnishings think carefully of any potential hazard

—Keep the room simple and not overstimulating visually or aurally. Display work at the back of the room, not in direct line of sight with blackboard and teacher

—Soft classical music as a background during quiet work can soothe children and adults

—Encourage discussion on health and ecological issues (particularly diet) so children on special diets are not regarded as freaks

—In cooking sessions try making healthy foods, eg: vegetable soup, instead of junk foods such as toffee!

—Support the parents and if you suspect they need outside help suggest local community resources

# CHAPTER TEN

# *Conclusion*

I very much hope that after reading this book, you do not see the issue of food/chemical sensitivity as just a problem for a few 'weak' individuals: Remember: 'it is not a question of who is sensitive, but how sensitive.' This is a problem that affects *everybody*.

Behavioural changes and symptoms due to sensitivities are an insidious warning that our bodies are not coping with the chemical concoction that we now live in and consume. Remember, behavioural changes occur before physical symptoms are obvious.

These subtle changes in behaviour and functional physical symptoms are fooling us into accepting aberrant behaviour and a compromised picture of health as normal. It is extremely worrying to hear even professionals accepting unprovoked or spontaneous severe aggressive outbursts as 'normal' in even very young children.

The profound effects that sensitivities can have on physical and mental health are alarming. Mental health is not just the absence of mental illness, but the ability to successfully cope with and adjust to whatever life happens to bring. The effects of sensitivities on intellectual development and social and emotional functioning can drastically affect a person's coping mechanisms.

Sensitivities are a *social problem*. We cannot

individually carve the air up into pieces that we each keep clean. The community cannot afford to have otherwise healthy people intermittently 'tripping out' or 'away with the fairies'.

The human cost is appalling, and the financial cost in lost productivity must be staggering.

Unfortunately, until the community at large recognises this problem, it is left to individuals to cope as best as they can.

In the absence of much hard scientific research, we can either choose to pretend there is no problem, or we can use a degree of commonsense and minimise the use of chemicals by using realistic alternatives.

This is not a time when individuals should opt out by waiting to be 'led'. Government and industry respond remarkably well to consumer pressure! For example, the boom in the 'health' food industry.

As individuals, every time we make a purchase in any store, we are making a statement and giving a clear message about the type of life we want. Whenever we shop, we can make a conscious decision to choose the least chemically hazardous option (be it clothes, cleaners, food, etc.) or demand that satisfactory alternatives be available.

Professionals are in an excellent position to encourage the general public to make less hazardous choices and to find satisfactory alternatives.

Government and industry must also show a greater respect for the long-term ecological view, rather than the short-term political or financial view.

Significant exposure to man-made chemicals and the escalating interactive effects of these chemicals has really only occurred since World War Two. We are now seeing the first generation of children born to parents who themselves grew up in such a chemical enviroment. If all these behavioural and physical effects have happened in one generation, and we don't start taking sensible precautions, then—God help the next!

# *Appendix*

## Useful contacts and publications

**The Allergy Association of Australia** (AAA) is a self-help group for allergy/sensitivity patients.

The AAA can give names of professionals, services and organisations in your area who are familiar with allergy and sensitivity problems.

The newsletter collates information from many other similar organisations in Australia and overseas.

Allergy Association of Australia
PO Box 298
Ringwood Vic 3134

**The Allergy Research Organisation Australia** (AROA) was founded by professionals and patients aware of the desperate need to raise funds for research.

Sensitivity patients, professionals, and families alarmed by this problem can do something constructive by joining AROA. Members receive a newsletter four times a year.

Allergy Research Organisation of Australia
PO Box 4022
University of Melbourne
Parkville Vic 3052

# Sources of special foods and products

Local health food stores now stock a large range of products (foods, filters, ionisers, etc.) suitable for patients with sensitivities and this is usually the most convenient place to go to first. Packaging in health food stores is often cellophane and glass rather than plastics. Also, as health food stores tend to be owner-operated they are usually very obliging and will make an effort to meet special needs.

For larger items (furnishings, beds, etc.) and for a wider range of air and water filters, the **Allergy Aid Centre** provides an excellent service. Patients have found that the staff have a very good understanding of the products sold, and products can also be bought by mail-order.

Allergy Aid Centre
Shop 57, 1st Floor Pran Central
325 Chapel street
Prahran Vic 3181
Phone: (03) 529 7348

# *Bibliography*


*A–Z of Chemicals in the Home*, Toxic and Hazardous Chemicals Committee of the Total Environmental Centre, Sydney, 1986.

Aigner T. G. et al., *The Effects of Physostigmine and Scopolamine on Behaviour and Neural Biology*, 1986; (45):81–87.

Atkinson, R. L., *Opioid Regulation of Food Intake and Body Weight in Humans*, Federation Proceedings, 1987 Jan; 46(1).

Atrens D. & Curthoys I., *The Neurosciences and Behaviour*, Academic Press, 1982.

*Australian Allergy Association Newsletter.*

Beck A. T. & Emery G., *Anxiety Disorders and Phobias*, Basic Books, 1979.

Bell I. R. & King D., *Psychological and Physiological Research Relevent to Clinical Ecology, Overview of Current Literature*, Clinical Ecology, 1982 Spring; 1(1).

Besedovsky H., Del Rey A. & Sorkin E., *'What do the Immune System and Brain know about Each Other?'*, Immunology To-day, 1983; 4(12).

Blalock, J. E. & Smith E. M., *A Complete Regulatory Loop between the Immune and Neuroendocrine Systems*, Federation Proceedings, 1985 Jan; 44(1) Pt. 1.

Bland J. Ed., *Medical Applications of Clinical Nutrition*, Keats, 1983.

Buist R., *Food Chemical Sensitivity*, Harper and Row, 1986.

Burns D. D., *Feeling Good*, Signet, 1980.

Calabress J. P. et al., *Depression, Immune Competence and Prostaglandins of the E Series*, Psychiatry Res., 17:41–47.

Carson R., *Silent Spring*, Penguin, 1962.

Cawcutt L. & Watson C., *Pesicides: The New Plague* FOE, Collinwood, 1984.

Chandra R. K., *Effect of Macro- and Micronutrient Deficiencies and Excesses on Immune Response*, Food Technology, 1985 Feb; p. 91.

Cheraskin E. & Ringdorf W., *Psychodietics*, Bantam, 1976.

Cohen M. R et al., *High-Dose Naloxone Influsions in Normals*, Arch. Gen Psychiatry, 1983 June; 40.

De Lisi L. E. et al., *Serum Immunoglobulin Concentrations in Patients Admitted to an Acute Psychiatric In-patient Service*, Br. J. Psychiatry, 1984; 145: 666–65.

*Depression Stress and Immunity*, Lancet, June 1987.

Egger J., Carter C. M., Graham P. J., Gumley D., Soothill J. F., *Controlled Trial of Oligoantigenic treatment in the Hyperkinetic Syndrome*, Lancet, 1985, March 9; 1(8428):540–5.

Ellis, *Reason and Emotion in Psychotherapy*, Citadel, 1962.

Forman R., *How to Control Your Allergies*, Larchimont, 1982.

Gold M. S. et al., *Antimanic, Antidepressent and Antipanic Effects of Opiates: Clinical Neuroanatomical and Biochemical Evidence*, Ann NY Acad Science, 1982.

Gold P. E., *Glucose Modulation of Memory Storage Processing*, Behavioural and Neural Biology, 45: 527–36.

Hansesen, *Additive Code Breaker*, Lothian, 1986.

Hall R. H., *Food for Nought: The Decline in Nutrition*, Vintage, 1976.

Henry J. L., *Role of Circulating Opioids in the Modulation of Pain*, Ann NY Acad Science, 1986; 467: 169–81.

Hoffer A. & Walker N., *Nutrients for Age Without Senility*, 1980.

Howett T. A. & Rees L. H., *Endogenous Opiod Peptides and Hypothalamo-Pituitary Function*, Ann. Rev. Physiol., 48: 527–36.

Jabubowski P. & Lange A., *The Assertive Option*, Research Press, 1979.

Jeffrey D. B. & Katz R. G., *Take It Off, Keep It Off*, Spectrum, 1977.

Jemmott, J. B. et al., *Psycho-social Factors, Immunological Medication and Human Susceptibility to Infectious Illnesses: How Much Do We Know?*, Psychol. Bull., 1984; 95: 78–108.

Journal International Clinical Nutrition Review.

Kastin A. J., Zadina J. E., Banks W. A., Graf M. V., *Misleading Concepts in the Field of Brain Peptides*, Peptides 1984; 5 Suppl 1: 249–53.

Kastin, A. J., Galina Z. H., Horvarth A., Olson R. D., *Some Principles in the Peptide Field*, J Allergy Clin Immunol, 1987 Jan; 79(1): 6–11.

Kielholz Ed., *Masked Depression*, Hans Huber, 1973.

King D. S., *Double Blind Food Challenges Affecting Sensitive Children's Behaviour and Heart Rate*, Invited Address, 92nd Annual Congress of A.Ps.A., Toronto, Canada.

King David S., *Can Allergic Exposure Provide Psychological Symptoms? A Double Blind Test*, Biol. Psychiatry, 1981 Jan; 16(1): 3–19.

Kramer G. W., Ebert M. H., Lake C. R., McKinney W. T., *Hypersensitivity to D-amphetamine Several Years after Early Social Deprivation in Rhesus Monkeys*, Psychopharmacology (Berlin), 1984; 82(3): 266–71.

Lehnert H., Reinstein D. K., Strowbridge B. W., Wurtman R. J., *Neurochemical and Behavioural Consequences of Acute Uncontrollable Stress: Effects of Dietary Tyrosine*, Brain Res, 1984 Jun 15; 303(2): 215–23.

Leibowitz S. F., *Brain Monoamines and Peptides: Role in the Control of Eating Behaviour*, Federation Proceedings, 1986 Apr; 45(5).

Leuine A. S. et al., *Critical Review: Neuropeptides as Regulators of Consummatory Behaviours*, J. Nutr., 1986; 116: 2067–2077.

Levine S. A. & Kidd P. M., *Antioxidant Adaption: A Unified Disease Theory*,, J. Orthom. Psychiatry, 14(1); 19–38.

Lewinsohm P. M. et al., *Control Your Depression*, Spectrum, 1978.

Long J. & Holaday J., *Blood Brain Barrier: Endogenous Modulation by Acheral-Cortical Function*, Science, 1985 Mar; 227.

Luria, A. R., *The Working Brain*, Penguin, 1973.

Mackerness R., *Chemical Victims*, Pan, 1980.

Mackerness R., *Not All in the Mind*, Pan, 1976.

Mandell M., *Five Day Allergy Relief Diet*, Pocket Books, New York, 1970.

Marks J., *A Guide to the Vitamins: Their Role in Health and Disease*, M.T.P., 1975.

Martinez J. L., De Graaf J. S., *Quaternary Naloxone Enhances Acquisition of a Discriminated Y-maze Escape and a one-way active avoidance task in mice*, Psychopharmacology (Berlin), 1985; 87(4): 410–3.

Meares A., *Relief Without Drugs*, Fontana, 1970.

Meares A., *The New Woman*, Fontana, 1974.

Meisenberg G., Simmons W. H., *Minireview: Peptides and the Blood-brain Barrier*, Life Science, 1983 Jun 6; 32(23): 2611–23.

Melville A. & Johnson C., *Cured to Death*, Angus & Robertson, 1983.

Meyer D. R., *The Cerebal Cortex: It's Roles in Memory Storage and Remembering*, Physiological Psychology, 1984; 12(2): 81–88.

Minchin M., *Food for Thought*, Alma/Unwin, 1982.

Minchin M., *Breast Feeding Matters*, Alma/Union, 1985.

Morgan B. & Morgan R., *Brain Food*, Michael Joseph, 1986.

Morley J. E. & Levine A. S., *The Pharmacology of Eating Behaviour*, Ann. Rev. Pharmacol., 25: 127–46.

Nutrition and Mental Health, Hearing Select Committee on Nutrition and Human Needs, United States Senate, 1980, Parker House.

Nutrition Reviews, Supplement 1986 May; 44.

Orbach S., *Fat Is a Feminist Issue*, Hamlyn, 1978.

Orbach S., *What Do Women Want?* Michael Joseph, 1984.

Pardridge W. M. & Frak H. J. L., *Mechanisms of Peptide Transport from Blood to Brain* in Muller & Macloud R. (Eds.), *Neuroendocrine Perspectives*, 1983; 2(3).

Pardridge W., *Blood-Brain Transport of Nutrients*, Federation Proceedings, 1986 Jun; 45(7).

Pfaffer C., *Zinc and other Micro-Nutrients*, Pivot, 1978.

Pfeiffer C. C., *Mental and Elemental Nutrients*, Keats, 1975.

Philpott W. H. et al., *Brain Allergies*, Keats, 1980.

Plotmkoff N. P. & Murgo A. J., *Enkephalins—Endorphins: Stress and the Immune System*, Federation Proceedings, 1985 Jan; 44(1): 91–122.

Progess in Neurobiology, 1987; 28: 1–54.

Randolph T. C. & Moss R. W., *Allergies*, Turnstone Press, 1981.

Regtop H., *Practical Concepts in the Regulation of the Immune System*, Lecture, 1980.

Roitt, Brostoff, Male, *Immunology*, Gower, 1985.

Russell R. W., Overstreet D. H., *Mechanisms Underlying Sensitivity to Organophosphorus Anticholinesterase Compounds*, Prog Neurobiol, 1987; 28(2): 97–129.

Russell R. & Singer G., *Behavioural Toxicology: The Emergence of a New Discipline in Australian Psychology*, Aust. Psychol., 1982 Jul; 17(2).

Safer D. J. & Allen R. P., *Hyperactive Children*, University Park Press, 1976.

Schauss A., *Diet, Crime and Delinquency*, Parker House, 1981.

Sedgwick H., *Stress and Counter Stress*, Sun, 1983.

Sicuteri F., *Natural Opioids in Migraine*, Advances in Neurology, 1982; 33: 65–73.

Siebert G., Gessner B., Klasser M., *Energy Supply of the Central Nervous System*, Bibl Nutr Dieta, 1986; (38): 1–26.

Smith M. J., *When I Say No I Feel Guilty*, Bantam, 1977.

Sunberg N. D., *Assessment of Persons*, Prentice-Hall, 1977.

Van-Tiggelen C. J. M. et al., *Vitamin B12 Levels of Cerebrospinal Fluid in Patients with Organic Mental Disorder*, Personal Communication.

Van-Tiggelen C. J. M., *Alzheimer's Disease/Alcohol Dementia: Association with Zinc Deficiency and Cerebral Vitamin B12 Deficiency*, J. Orthom. Psychiatry 14(2); 97–104.

Van Tiggelen C. J. M., *Psychogeriatrics*, Aust. Family Physician, 1985 14(2).

Van Tiggelen C. J. M., *Disturbed Behaviour in the Elderly*, Aust. Family Physician, 1986 15(2).

Van Tiggelen C. J. M., *Trace Elements, Microsomal Liver Enzyme Induction and Amino Acids: A New Perspective in Biological Psychiatry*, Trace element—Analytical Chemistry in Medicine and Biology 1987 4; 419–431 Editors: P. Bratter, P. Schamel, W. De Gruyter & Co. Berlin—New York.

Walsh K., *Neuropsychology*, Churchhill-Livingstone, 1978.

Wingfield, Symes, *The Psychology of Human Memory*, Academic Press, 1981.

Williams C. A., Schupf N., *The Neuropharmacology of Immune Complex Activity in the Rat Hypothalamous*, Ann NY Acad Sci, 1987; 496: 250–63.

Wittersheim G. et al., *Mental Task-Induced Strain and Its After Effect Assessed through Variations in Plasma Cortisol Levels*, Biol. Psychol., 1985; 21: 123–132.